Planning Australia's Healthy Built Environments

Planning Australia's Healthy Built Environments shines a quintessentially Australian light on the links between land use planning and human health. A burgeoning body of empirical research demonstrates the ways urban structure and governance influence human health—and Australia is playing a pivotal role in developing understandings of the relationships between health and the built environment.

This book takes a retrospective look at many of the challenges faced in pushing the healthy built environment agenda forward. It provides a clear and theoretically sound framework to inform this work into the future. With an emphasis on context and the pursuit of equity, Jennifer L. Kent and Susan Thompson supply specific ways to better incorporate idiosyncrasies of place and culture into urban planning interventions for health promotion.

By chronicling the ways health and the built environment scholarship and practice can work together, *Planning Australia's Healthy Built Environments* enters into new theoretical and practical debates in this critically important area of research. This book will resonate with both health and built environment scholars and practitioners working to create sustainable and health-supportive urban environments.

Jennifer L. Kent is a Research Fellow in the School of Architecture, Design and Planning at the University of Sydney. Jennifer's research interests are at the intersections between urban planning, transport and health. She publishes regularly in high-ranking scholarly journals, and her work is used to inform policy in Australia. Prior to commencing a career in academia, she worked as a planner both for government and as a consultant.

Susan Thompson is Professor of Planning in the Faculty of the Built Environment at The University of New South Wales. Susan's academic career encompasses research and teaching in social and cultural planning, qualitative research methodologies and healthy built environments. She has received numerous awards for her contributions to urban planning in Australia, including the Sidney Luker Memorial Medal in 2015 and the Australian Urban Research Medal in 2017.

Routledge Research in Planning and Urban Design

Routledge Research in Planning and Urban Design is a series of academic monographs for scholars working in these disciplines and the overlaps between them. Building on Routledge's history of academic rigour and cutting-edge research, the series contributes to the rapidly expanding literature in all areas of planning and urban design.

Social Economics and the Solidarity City
Brendan Murtagh

Participatory Design Theory
Using Technology and Social Media to Foster Civic Engagement
Edited by Oswald Devisch, Liesbeth Huybrechts, Roel De Ridder

Evolving Public Space in South Africa
Towards Regenerative Space in the Post-Apartheid City
Karina Landman

Post Socialist Urban Infrastructures
Edited by Tauri Tuvikene, Wladimir Sgibnev, Carola S. Neugebauer

The Metaphysical City
Six Ways of Understanding the Urban Milieu
Rob Sullivan

The City in Geography
Renaturing the Built Environment
Benedict Anderson

Public Infrastructure, Private Finance
Developer Obligations and Responsibilities
Edited by Demetrio Muñoz Gielen and Erwin van der Krabben

www.routledge.com/Routledge-Research-in-Planning-and-Urban-Design/book-series/RRPUD

Planning Australia's Healthy Built Environments

Jennifer L. Kent and
Susan Thompson

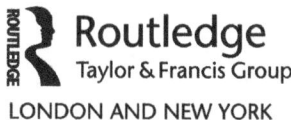

Routledge
Taylor & Francis Group

LONDON AND NEW YORK

First published 2019
by Routledge

2 Park Square, Milton Park, Abingdon, Oxfordshire OX14 4RN
52 Vanderbilt Avenue, New York, NY 10017

Routledge is an imprint of the Taylor & Francis Group, an informa business

First issued in paperback 2020

Library of Congress Cataloging-in-Publication Data
Names: Kent, Jennifer, 1951– author. | Thompson, Susan,
    1954– author.
Title: Planning Australia's healthy built environments / Jennifer
    L. Kent and Susan Thompson.
Description: New York : Routledge, 2019. |
    Series: Routledge research in planning and urban design |
    Includes bibliographical references.
Identifiers: LCCN 2018052936 (print) | LCCN
    2018053015 (ebook) | ISBN 9781315524573 (e-book) |
    ISBN 9781138696365 (hardback)
Subjects: LCSH: City planning—Health aspects—Australia. |
    Urban health—Australia.
Classification: LCC RA566.5.A8 (ebook) | LCC RA566.5.A8 K46
    2019 (print) | DDC 362.1/0420994—dc23
LC record available at https://lccn.loc.gov/2018052936

ISBN: 978-1-138-69636-5 (hbk)
ISBN: 978-0-367-67092-4 (pbk)

Typeset in Sabon
by Apex CoVantage, LLC

Jennifer: For John Manefield and Jorie Ryan
Susan: For Ruth Lyla Micheli Thompson

We respectfully acknowledge the traditional custodians of Australia—the Indigenous peoples who have inhabited this land for millennia. They are a living part of the oldest continuous existing culture on earth. We acknowledge all Aboriginal and Torres Strait Islander Elders, past and present and their communities who have been stewards of the places that all people in Australia now enjoy.

Contents

Figures

Tables

Boxes

Acknowledgements

Tangible work on this book began on a wintry July morning when Jennifer and Susan sat together in the Hawthorne Canal dog park to discuss the project. Many co and solo working sessions ensued to produce *Planning Australia's Healthy Built Environments*.

Although the dog park hosted the first discussion about the specifics of the book, in reality its contents are the culmination of a working relationship that has spanned a decade. We are first, therefore, thankful to Routledge for giving us the opportunity to put into words many of the concepts and practices that have fuelled our curiosities, conversations, teaching and research over the years.

In developing the text specifically, we would like to thank the many colleagues Australia wide, students, friends and research study participants, who have helped refine our understandings of the links between health and urban planning. In addition, several people have provided direct assistance to bring the book into being. Particular thanks to Laura Goh and Victoria McRae for research assistance, Jason Harrison for bibliographic checking, Alison Kent for meticulous proofreading and Homa Rahmat for developing our ideas into infographics. Chris Stevens and Jorie Ryan provided invaluable assistance with photography. Various others have commented on draft components of the book. Particular thanks to Michelle Daley, Martin Karm, Paul Klarenaar, Peter Sainsbury, Tony Capon and Hugh MacKay.

Jennifer acknowledges the support of colleagues and friends at the School of Architecture, Design and Planning, University of Sydney, particularly Robyn Dowling and Nicole Gurran. Any text of hers must recognise the joy and distraction provided by companion cats, Rusty and Audrey, and Olive, the sausage dog. Nash, of course, has also provided love, distraction and care, and his uncanny knack for 'keeping it real' is cherished.

Susan acknowledges financial support for the publication from her Faculty–Built Environment at UNSW, Sydney. Special thanks to her many students, Peter McCue, practitioner colleague, for healthy planning inspiration over the years and Nick Chapman for his inspiring dedication and commitment to sustainable, healthy places. Thanks to Lennie, furry feline companion, and to David, soulmate and never-failing supporter.

Abbreviations

ABC	Australian Broadcasting Corporation
ABS	Australia Bureau of Statistics
ACT	Australian Capital Territory
AHURI	Australasian Housing and Urban Research Institute
ALGA	Australian Local Government Association
AIHW	Australian Institute of Health and Welfare
AMA	Australian Medical Association
BITRE	Bureau of Infrastructure, Transport and Regional Economics
CPTED	Crime Prevention Through Environmental Design
DALY	Disability-Adjusted Life Year
DCP	Development Control Plan
EBM	Evidence Based Medicine
HILDA	Household, Income and Labour Dynamics in Australia
NCC	National Construction Code
NHMRC	National Health and Medical Research Council
NSW	New South Wales
NT	Northern Territory
OECD	Organization for Economic Co-operation and Development
PIA	Planning Institute of Australia
RACP	Royal Australian College of Physicians
RSPCA	Royal Society for the Protection of Animals
SA	South Australia
SEIFA	Socio-Economic Indexes for Areas
TAS	Tasmania
UN	United Nations
UNSW	The University of New South Wales
VIC	Victoria
VKT	Vehicle Kilometres Travelled
WA	Western Australia
WHO	World Health Organization
WSUD	Water Sensitive Urban Design

Introduction

Any text with a focus on the people and places of Australia must start with acknowledgement of Australia's recent history.

Proclaimed a British colony in 1788, Australia is often inaccurately labelled a relatively young country. Yet, at the time of the British invasion, Australia was populated by the oldest living culture in the world: that of the Aboriginal and Torres Strait Islander people. This is a culture that goes back at least 60,000 years, adapting over time to exist in relative harmony with Australia's harsh biophysical environment.

This existence was utterly destroyed by British colonisation. In 1788, the best estimates suggest that there were approximately 750,000 Aboriginal and Torres Strait Islander people organised into over 500 nations across the land mass now known as Australia. By 1900, introduced disease, disenfranchisement from land, and violent conflict with colonisers had reduced this population by 90%. At the time of Australia's 2016 census, there were just under 650,000 people identifying as Aboriginal or Torres Strait Islander, comprising 2.8% of the total population. Sadly, the legacy of ill-treatment and poor health has continued through the 20th Century, with today's Aboriginal and Torres Strait Islander population continuing to experience poor health outcomes relative to the rest of the nation.

Modern Australia continues to grapple with the process of acknowledging, understanding and redressing the implications of British colonisation. Key to this is the tacit acceptance that our nation is born out of a shameful, and relatively recent, legacy of invasion and ill-treatment. It is from this position that Australia comes to the task of living in harmony both with each other and the fragile biophysical land that supports us. In modern Australia, this is a task of grand reconciliation—of diverse cultures, the unrelenting demands of modern life, a market-driven system of distribution and increased awareness of risk, safety and each other. Urban planning, as a well-honed practice of systematic compromise, is integral to this challenge.

Conceptualising Urban Planning

What exactly is urban planning? We are urban planners—a 'fact' proclaimed by multiple 'labels'. For example, we both have experience working under that job title. It is the name attributed to components of our tertiary studies. And now, of course, it is a descriptor used to define our contribution to the university system. We realise these labels do not provide a definition. However, the desire to define urban planning has been the subject of many debates, both theoretical and practical, and we do not wish to complicate them further here. As a text with a distinct intention to be practical, we are more interested in what it is that planners in Australia actually do.

Urban planning was first recognised as a state obligation in Australia during the nation's first experience of rapid urbanisation in the late 19th Century. It was out of this upheaval that planning emerged as a tool for reform, broadly based on a set of goals to improve housing, sanitation and amenity, to raise living and working standards and to make people "cheerful, hopeful and healthy" (Garnaut 2000, p. 47). This is a relatively optimistic aspiration. As modern-day planners, we feel compelled to reveal that the reality of planning in contemporary Australia is much more reactive.

We mentioned above that planning's power is in the process of guiding systematic compromise. By this, we mean that planners do not operate above, or aside from, the cultural, political, economic and environmental systems and processes that drive contemporary Australian society. In particular, if a subset of political and economic elements is supportive of a proposed urban process or outcome, planners often have little choice but to accept the bulk of it. This is not a position of complete disempowerment. In fact, because we are at the centre of realising these visions, the reality is often to the contrary. Urban planners in Australia are granted opportunities to strategically promote outcomes that we, as professionals, know are more sustainable and healthier.

In a very practical sense, we do this in multiple matters pertaining to land use. We seek ways to ethically and sustainably distribute housing relative to other uses, such as employment lands, open space, services (including schools, hospitals, community facilities and everything in between) and infrastructure delivery. We understand the links between these things—ensuring efficient and effective networks of transport and technology are key urban challenges we embrace. Add to this the need to manage these factors in the economic, political, cultural and environmental milieu mentioned above, and one can see how a discipline is formed. In this text, we call this discipline 'urban planning'.

These are the structures and processes that concern planners, but to what end? It is at this point that health, as a fundamental aim of planning, can shine as a key concept. Truth be told, as planners, we would prefer a more nuanced description of what drives urban planning in Australia. One that explicitly incorporates notions of equity, ethics, respect, authenticity, trust and even a modicum of fun. Yet better human health as a goal of urban planning is a more simple, powerful and seductive concept—one that can easily be applied to steer the ship of political economy. It is an easily interpretable embodiment of these more complex aims.

Conceptualising Health

And what of health? Efforts to define health have been just as resolute, and at times circumscribed, as those seeking to define urban planning. We are compelled to adopt the widely accepted view of the World Health Organization, which positions health as "a complete state of mental, physical and social wellbeing and more than just the presence or absence of disease" (World Health Organization 1948, p. 1). We add that in this 21st Century world, a healthy individual must also have a degree of autonomy and adaptability—the capacity to withstand transition (Canguilhem 1943). Recalling our intention to be practical, what does this actually mean? In addition to our biophysical make-up, and the good or bad habits we pick up, our health is also influenced by the social, economic and biophysical environments in which we find ourselves. These are known as the 'social determinants of health'. This is a concept that is key to this book, and its composition and application are covered in Chapter 2—Australia's Health. For now, what is relevant is that a person's health is as much shaped by contextual factors as it is dependent upon individual and behavioural factors. Health cannot be extracted from things such as access to education, the location and security of the home, type and permanency of employment, and access to opportunities for recreation, socialisation, healthy food preparation and other practices of self-care. In this way of thinking about health, a role for urban planning seems obvious. Urban planners are the ones guiding decisions on the environments that influence the social determinants of health—hence the emergence of the concept of healthy planning and the need for a text on planning Australia's healthy built environments.

Conceptualising Healthy Built Environments

Having outlined the theoretical space in which planning and health come together, we are left with the need to conceptualise the desired outcome of this convergence. What do we mean by a 'healthy built environment'?

Principally, a healthy built environment is one that has a positive impact on health. It is a place where the streets, neighbourhoods, workplaces, transport and food distribution systems enable people to lead physically and mentally healthy lives, fulfil their potential and be resilient to adversity. Healthy built environments are also equitable and diverse environments, where all members of society have fair access to the health-promoting benefits of place.

A healthy built environment is characterised by a mix of people, infrastructure, design and distribution. At the scale of the city, healthy built environments require connectivity through active and public transport infrastructure, dense networks of green and public spaces and a diversity of housing choices. Healthy cities aspire to the strategic location of services and employment in centres close to where people live so that the things people need to be healthy can be accessed easily and safely. They typically discourage over-reliance on the private car. At the scale of the neighbourhood, healthy built environments contain intuitive street networks that are safe and public and open spaces that are responsive to context and well maintained. Healthy neighbourhoods provide infrastructure for community interaction and physical activity, such as playgrounds, public squares, community facilities and parks. They offer a diversity of densities and uses, catering to the needs of different populations. At the scale of the building, healthy built environments are designed to provide protection from harms, including noise and fumes and extremes of heat and cold. They are well constructed to ensure longevity and resilience. Healthy buildings are open to the streets on which they sit. They encourage social interactions but also provide spaces of privacy and retreat. At all scales, healthy built environments are planned and managed to be inclusive and responsive to diverse spatial, temporal and cultural contexts. Planning for healthy built environments aspires to equity and balance in built, social and economic outcomes.

These three conceptualisations—urban planning, health and healthy built environments—are foundations for the explorations, ideas and evidence presented throughout this book.

About This Book

The book is structured in three parts that are brought together in a final chapter—Reflections on Principles of Healthy Planning. Part I is a succinct tour of a series of indicators, concepts, systems and structures relevant to Australian planning and Australia's health. We etch out the theoretical and practical spaces that host the link between health and urban planning in Australia and discuss key challenges. This Part also includes a timeline of the development of interest in, and action on, healthy built environments in Australia.

Part II introduces four 'Domains of Wellbeing'. These domains are comprised of three behaviours (physical activity, social interaction and healthy eating) and one critical realm—a healthy planet. Our rationale for these domains is that they are all linked to risk factors that are commonly implicated in many of the diseases that challenge modern Australia. Most obviously, these risk factors are physical inactivity, social isolation and unhealthy eating. Taking a fresh perspective on the typical risks explored in this space, we also position an unhealthy planet as a risk factor for human health.

Part III identifies four 'Domains of the Built Environment'. These are the planning structures and systems that can be modified to promote health. We traverse several built domains that are integral to modern life: home, transport, healthcare, employment, education and the public realm. For each, we paint a picture of the way these domains can promote health, exploring strategies for their actualisation within the constraints of the systems that govern land use in Australia.

Some final notes on the style and substance of this book: Firstly, where possible, we have tried to use examples from Australia. This does not mean our recommendations and reflections do not apply to other countries experiencing similar health and planning challenges. We recognise that many of the standards, processes and practices we describe as Australian are common internationally; however, for the sake of simplicity, we have not always acknowledged this.

Secondly, our focus is primarily on metropolitan areas. This comes from the reality that most Australians live in large metropolitan cities. While both the health problems and environments experienced in rural and regional Australia are unique, many of the concepts covered apply to any place in Australia that is 'built-up'. This includes the regional centres and country towns that comprise home for those living outside major cities. Related to this is the fact that readers should not be distracted by the term 'built environment'. By this, we simply mean environments that have been modified by human intervention, and at times we interchange the term for urban environments. Similarly, we employ the terms 'urban planning', 'land use planning' and sometimes simply 'planning' to describe the processes of managing built environments. This is reflective of practice in Australia.

Thirdly, our ideas are our own. However, we are incredibly lucky to be able to draw on the research, policy, experiences and accepted wisdom of the professionals with whom we work to form these ideas. Again, for the sake of clarity, we have intentionally limited the use of citations and references within our text. This book is not intended to be a review of the literature—there are many such reviews in existence. Instead, the intention is to draw together frameworks, reflections, ideas and practices as a way to discuss healthy built environments in Australia. Readers can be assured that this organic synthesis is evidence-based.

Finally, a note on the way this text came to be. We feel it is important to acknowledge that Jennifer has written the bulk of the words, and through this writing process she has developed the book's structure. Susan has provided the invaluable safety net of detailed edits and has been a vital filter for ideas and insights. The ideas in this book are the product of years of working together on an area of interest that started as a result of Susan forging ground, from an urban planning perspective, in the healthy built environments space in Australia.

This is our contribution to the journey of planning Australia's healthy built environments. It is our hope that this book inspires others to join us and those already along for the ride to keep travelling.

References

Canguilhem, G. (1943) *The Normal and the Pathological*, Zone Books, New York.

Garnaut, C. (2000) Towards metropolitan organisation: Town planning and the garden city idea, in Hamnett, S. and Freestone, R. eds., *The Australian Metropolis: A Planning History*, Routledge, New York.

World Health Organization (1948) *Constitution of the World Health Organization*, World Health Organization, Geneva.

Part I

Introducing Australia

1 Australia and Australia's Planning

Introduction

What is it about Australia?

Many words have been written, many studies done and many syntheses completed about the links between health and urban planning. What is it about Australia that demands an entire text dedicated to this relationship in this country?

We all come to modern life with different histories, experiences, expectations and ways of doing, knowing and being. In reality, to map a boundary around a group of people based on the geography of where they live is artificial, and increasingly so in our connected world. Some would even argue it is against the grain of a common mantra throughout this book: to respect the nuances of context. But boundaries do exist, creating groups of people who, at some stage and at some level, call Australia home. Some of the boundaries are solid and the result of tangible entities, such as governance, law and, of course, geography. Others are less concrete, created by cultural heritage, experience, knowledge and practices. It is all of these characteristics that draw us together (and pull us apart) to shape what we believe is a quintessentially Australian approach to the challenge of healthy built environments.

This chapter provides an introduction to Australia's demography, population geography and governance, including the governance of urban planning.

A Brief Social and Demographic Profile of Australia

Australia is a vast land mass with a diverse population. We are organised into six States and two Territories. The capital cities of these States and Territories are home to the majority of Australia's inhabitants, and the population is overwhelmingly concentrated around the coastal fringe.

The Australian Census of Population and Housing is the most reliable source of social and demographic data in Australia. Conducted every five years, it allows us to develop a basic narrative about the social and

Table 1.1 Australia's population

State	Total population (24.3 million)	Capital city	% of State population living in State capital city
New South Wales	7,798,000	Sydney	65
Victoria	6,244,000	Melbourne	77
Queensland	4,884,000	Brisbane	49
Western Australia	2,568,000	Perth	79
South Australia	1,717,000	Adelaide	77
Tasmania	519,000	Hobart	44
Australian Capital Territory	406,000	Canberra	100
Northern Territory	245,000	Darwin	40

Source: Australian Bureau of Statistics 2017

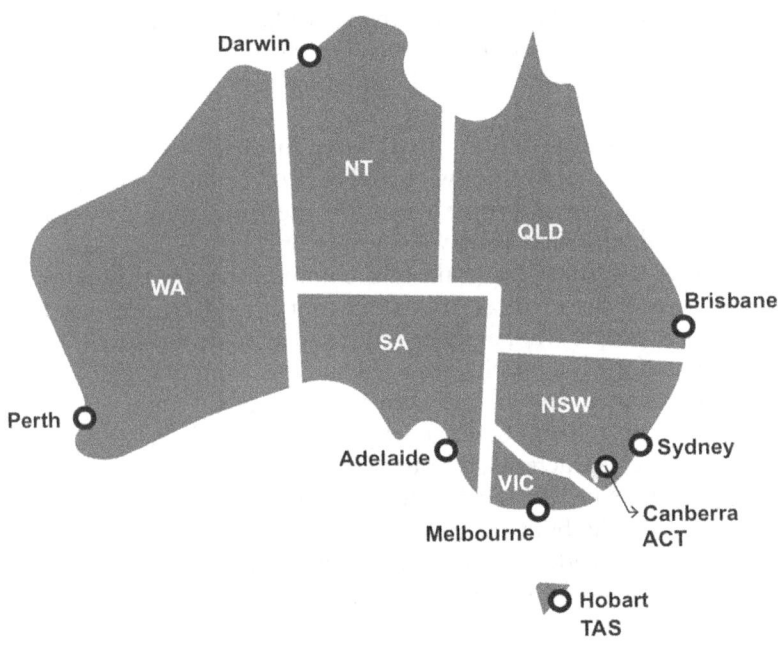

Figure 1.1 Australia's six States, two Territories and capital cities

demographic characteristics of the Australian population. The count is managed by a government agency known as the Australian Bureau of Statistics (ABS). It is a fundamental tool for informing better understandings of Australia's challenges and opportunities. Its completion on 'census night' is compulsory. Questions are asked about age, gender, incomes, occupations, dwelling types and occupancy, ancestry, languages spoken, transportation modes and optional questions, such as religious affiliation.

The most recent Australian census was held in August 2016. At that time, the population of Australia was estimated at 24.3 million, an increase of 1.87 million since 2011. This is a growth rate of 1.6% per year, slightly less than the 1.8% per year growth experienced between 2006 and 2011. Over this period, the States of Victoria and New South Wales contributed 60% to Australia's population increase compared with just 42% between 2006 and 2011. This indicates population growth in Australia is increasingly concentrated in the two States that are already the nation's largest.

This growth has two components: natural increase (the number of births minus the number of deaths) and net overseas migration. In 2016, the contribution to population growth was higher from net overseas migration (55.2%) than from natural increase (44.8%). At that time, 26.3% of the Australian population was born overseas, and 17.9% came from non-English–speaking backgrounds. Of note is that the backgrounds of our migrant populations are changing as we continue to experience increased migration from Asian countries, particularly China, India and the Philippines, and less migration from European countries, such as Italy and Greece, and the United Kingdom. Migrant groups are mostly choosing to settle in cities, which generally offer greater access to skilled jobs and a range of educational opportunities. In 2016, 94% of Chinese and Indian-born residents lived in our capital cities, with 75% choosing either Sydney or Melbourne. Representative of the fact that we remain a constitutional monarchy under the reign of the Queen of England, in 2016, the majority of migrants living in Australia came from the United Kingdom. This trend has endured since it started with the British invasion in 1788.

Table 1.2 Top 10 birthplaces of people born overseas, 2016

In 2016, 26.3% of the Australian population was born overseas. The following are the top ten birthplaces of people born overseas:

	Birthplace	*Percentage of Australia's population*
1.	United Kingdom	4.6%
2.	New Zealand	2.2%
3.	China	2.2%
4.	India	1.9%
5.	Philippines	1.0%
6.	Vietnam	0.9%
7.	Italy	0.7%
8.	South Africa	0.7%
9.	Malaysia	0.6%
10.	Sri Lanka	0.5%

Source: Australian Bureau of Statistics 2017

An Ageing Population?

We often consider that Australia's population is ageing. However, analyses of the age structure of the population over the last three Censuses from 2006, 2011 and 2016 indicate a series of additional shifts in the age of Australians over the last decade. There is the progression of the 'baby boomer' generation (a term used to reference the large natural increase in Australia's population experienced after World War II) from middle to older age. In particular, Australia has experienced strong growth of people aged 65–74 years. As this generation moves through the age spectrum, they will continue to shape policy, particularly around housing and the provision of healthcare. We have also experienced rapid growth of the young adult population (20–34 years) and the child population (0–10 years). These trends are the result of a notable shift in Australian population dynamics around the turn of the Millennium. During this period, Australia saw a reversal in what had become a long-running trend of declining fertility rates (Alexander 2017). Perhaps more influential, however, is that Australia also experienced a spike in migration that coincided with the Global Financial Crisis of 2008. With the Australian economy the 'envy of the world' throughout the Global Financial Crisis, Australia became an attractive destination for foreigners, and many Australians living overseas repatriated (Deacon 2016). Accordingly, in 2008, migration surged, exceeding 300,000 persons in 2009—a figure double the previous peaks.

Equality in Australia

Equality is a theme that arises often throughout this book, primarily because of the undeniable and evidence-based links between equality and health. The equality of a nation can be measured in multiple ways. We are particularly interested in the concentration of indicators of disadvantage in Australia and the gaps between the wealthiest and poorest Australians relative to other Organization for Economic Co-operation and Development (OECD) countries.

The distribution of disadvantage in Australia is measured by the Socio-Economic Indexes for Areas (SEIFA). This is an index maintained by the ABS, informed by data from the Census and applied to various geographical scales. It incorporates things such as:

- Percentage of low-income households
- Unemployment rate
- Percentage of low-skilled occupations and people without qualifications
- Percentage of households without a car
- Percentage of people living in overcrowded dwellings

- Percentage of people under 70 with a disability
- Percentage of children with jobless parents
- Percentage of people with poor English proficiency

SEIFA scores are expressed on a scale where lower numbers always mean more disadvantage and less advantage, while higher numbers mean less disadvantage and more advantage. They are standardised so that the average for Australia is always close to 1,000.

From the 2016 Census, the top ten least disadvantaged areas were all located in Sydney's northern suburbs and the western suburbs of Perth. The ten most extremely disadvantaged areas were all concentrated in remote Indigenous communities in Queensland and the Northern Territory. Indigenous status is not included as one of the characteristics in the SEIFA index. The main drivers of this extreme level of disadvantage in these communities are low incomes, overcrowded dwellings and low education levels. While these outliers mask general trends, in summary, disadvantage in Australia is overwhelmingly concentrated in rural and regional areas, and populations in our cities display lower levels of disadvantage. There are, however, substantial pockets of disadvantage in Australian cities. Indeed, the socio-economic gaps between urban areas with concentrations of wealth and concentrations of disadvantage are widening. The distribution of this disadvantage does have a distinctly Australian pattern—wealth is generally clustered in inner urban areas of cities, and disadvantage is distributed through suburban and outer urban communities.

Other measures of equality assess the gap between rich and poor—which can be done on a national scale—to facilitate international comparisons. The distribution of measures such as gross national income, household disposable income, adult education level, and employment rate exposes this gap. To demonstrate the degree of equality in Australia relative to other OECD nations, we concentrate on income. Income is defined as household disposable income in a particular year. Income inequality among countries can be measured by several indicators, including the oft-cited Gini coefficient. This is a measure of statistical dispersion, which is based on the comparison of cumulative proportions of the population against cumulative proportions of income they receive. Much of the recent debate surrounding inequality has focused on top earners, especially the 'top 1%', and over-reliance on the Gini coefficient perpetuates this. The relative decline of low earners and low-income households in a nation is less examined—not just the bottom 10% but the lowest 40%. The Palma ratio can be used to measure this. The higher the ratio, the higher the level of income concentration, or income inequality, in a country. The latest figures available (from 2014) indicate that Australia's Palma ratio is 1.3 (OECD 2018). This ranks Australia 11th of the 35 OECD countries. Figure 1.2 shows Australia's

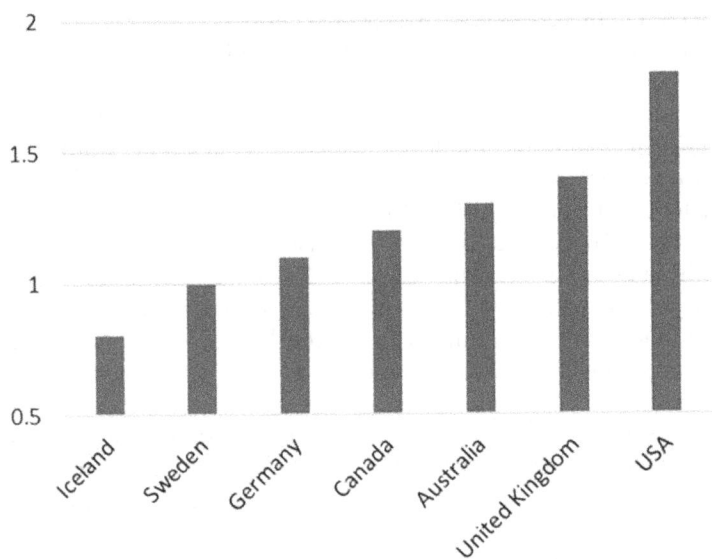

Figure 1.2 Palma ratio for selected OECD countries, including Australia
Source: OECD 2018

Palma ratio relative to several other OECD countries. A disturbing trend, with inevitable impacts on people's health, is that most indicators suggest that Australia is becoming an increasingly inequitable country. This ominous fact has been explored by many scholars (see Leigh 2013 for an interesting review).

Where Do We Live? Australia's Population Geography

An Urban Nation

The cultural subtext of Australia's historical national identity is defined by the bush, desert and 'outback'. These places are generally depicted as vast tracts of arid and dangerous wilderness. From Dorothy McKellar's 'land of sweeping plains' to Paul Hogan's personification of Mick 'Crocodile' Dundee, it seems we like to portray ourselves as a desert-dwelling nation of pioneers, doing it tough in the wilds of a perilous and untamed land. The reality, however, is quite different. Since British invasion in 1788, Australia has housed a highly urbanised and coastal population, with most of us living in cities and larger towns less than 50 kilometres from the ocean. There is a swathe of contemporary reasons for this, ranging from our settlement history—based on the need to locate close to sea ports for trade—to the current concentration of labour markets and other fiscal functions in existing cities. The primary reason for our coastal concentration, however, is that much of our nation's interior is simply uninhabitable. The availability of water is a key component of this. Australia comprises a land area of about 7.692 million square kilometres, yet 20% of this is officially classified as desert. Over 35% of the Australian continent receives so little rain that it is also effectively desert. As well as having a low average annual rainfall, rainfall across Australia is incredibly variable from place to place and season to season. Temperatures range from highs of 50 degrees Celsius in the central desert to below freezing in the higher regions of the country's southeast. Although we have some mountainous areas, Australia is generally a very flat continent, ensuring our major rivers are slow-flowing. Adding to the general inhabitability of much of the continent, thick regolith blankets the vast areas of the interior. This is a dusty and rocky surface, vulnerable to erosion through both wind and water processes. It is unsuitable for most high-yield crops and easily compacted by the hard hooves of many traditionally farmed animals, such as cattle and sheep. This climatic variability and geological character make the majority of the Australian land mass incredibly fragile. The native plants and animals, and the Indigenous peoples of Australia, have all adapted over thousands of years to accommodate and live in synthesis with this fragility. But the comforts and speed characterising our modern lives would simply not survive. As a result, our population generally concentrates around the more temperate and arable environments of our coasts and immediate hinterlands.

Linked to the coastal concentration of our population, at the time of the 2016 Census, over 90% of the population lived in 'urban' regions. Urban here is defined as built-up areas of towns and cities of more than 1,000 people. Over 67% of the population live in one of Australia's eight largest cities, and 58% live in just the top two—Sydney and Melbourne (see Table 1.1). Australians, therefore, tend to congregate in larger cities, and this tendency towards centralisation is increasing over time. Nationally, over the five years between 2011 and 2016, 76% of population growth occurred in greater capital city areas. Although there is an emergent pattern of internal migration from capital cities to smaller regional centres, it is more than offset by the arrival of overseas migrants, who tend to choose the major cities as their first Australian home.

The Structure of Australian Cities

As a highly urbanised nation, the various built, political and economic structures shaping Australia's cities provide the foundations for healthy built environments. Transport systems, the density of uses, the location of shops, offices and services relative to housing, and the provision of open space and community facilities, are particularly relevant. The way these things impact upon health—and are planned in Australia—is the subject of this entire book! The following section seeks to provide a basic rundown of some of the structures and processes within Australian urban areas, giving some insight as to how these came about.

By global standards, the predominant urban form in Australian cities is low-density. Aside from some inner urban areas in our major cities, detached dwellings have dominated the residential landscape. The suburbs of our cities are characterised by relatively large houses located on generous allotments, separated by substantial setbacks, with each block's territory firmly demarcated by a fence. Employment opportunities have been scattered in a rather haphazard way across each metropolis, with most cities retaining a strong central business district that continues to host many of the places where people who live in the suburbs work. This pattern of development is commonly termed 'urban sprawl'. It is a legacy of Australian cities that ensures car use dominates daily transport practices, private backyards take precedence over the provision of public open space, and retail uses are often centralised in large shopping precincts that are not necessarily close to homes or supportive of local economies. These suburbs can be places where contact with neighbours is inhibited by streets that discourage walking, dwellings are closed off from the street and, often, a distinct cultural appreciation of privacy and space exists.

To understand just how deep-seated the Australian attachment to lower-density living is, it is important to examine the historical development of its urban areas. In short, our lower-density urban landscapes are the result of a confluence of government policy, economic change, demographic shifts and consumer demand, the foundations of which can be seen as early as the 19th Century. It was not until the mid-19th Century that Australian cities started to grow beyond the confines of central areas. Unlike the United Kingdom, Europe and, to an extent, North America, this meant that our cities developed after the Industrial Revolution. As a result, the crowded inner city slums, which often accompanied the burgeoning business of industrial manufacturing, could generally be avoided. Instead, early forms of public transport enabled Australia's growing urban populations to spread well beyond the boundaries of main commercial areas. People built out in wedges of escape to the suburbs, and this trend enshrined the separation of employment and residential uses that still defines Australian cities. Into the late 1800s, a boom period led to an increase in general popular wealth, and the availability of cheap and abundant land provided many Australian families with the opportunity to own their own home. Further expansion of public transport networks meant that these homes did not need to be within walking distance of workplaces. As a result, by the time of Australia's Federation in 1901, Australian cities were already characterised by low-density residential urban form and long distances between uses. This structure continued to be reinforced throughout the 20th Century.

At the beginning of the 1900s, an influx of investment from Europe coincided with a Federal government push to promote manufacturing as a source of jobs for Australia's growing population. The resultant new industries represented employment opportunities for the existing population and attracted swathes of international migrants. This basically ensured city-dwellers had jobs and were not tempted to leave the metropolis for an often hard and unpredictable life in fledgling regional communities. Concurrently, several developments occurred in transport technology. The electrification of trams and trains meant that the growing population could continue to disperse outwards from the city core in search of the suburbs, yet remain connected to the city and other pockets of employment (Hamnett and Freestone 2000).

It was from this dispersed urban fabric that a series of economic, demographic and technological changes occurred to produce the era of the 'long boom' associated with the 1950s and '60s. The impact of this period of economic, demographic, social and technological change on urban Australia cannot be underestimated. Politically, the era was one of relative stability, with a single party and Prime Minister (Robert Menzies) retaining office from 1949 to 1966. It was a time of economic prosperity and unprecedented population growth, again resulting from immigration and a baby boom. In the 24 years between the 1947 and 1971 Censuses, the populations of Australia's five largest cities almost doubled from four to eight million (Forster 2006). Home ownership, epitomised by the 'quarter-acre block' with its detached dwelling and ample (private) backyard, was reinforced as the desired residential tenure, soon becoming a tacit expectation, accessible to anyone who worked hard enough. To accommodate this new and optimistic population, housing, planning and transport policies continued to provide suburbs for low-density detached dwellings on larger blocks, which were increasingly longer distances from places of employment. Any issues associated with this approach were thought to be resolved with the onset of private car use as an accessible form of transport. It was during this time that the cost of purchasing a private car was substantially reduced, bringing the freedom, autonomy and privacy of driving within the reach of most families. The government responded by investing in road infrastructure rather than maintaining or expanding public transport networks. This ensured the car became not only the transport mode of choice in Australia's cities but also a necessity.

By the 1980s, demographic shifts, increasingly long commutes, emergent popular concern for environmental issues, and a nascent cultural shift away from suburban living prompted State governments across Australia to entertain the pursuit of a compact city. This approach advocated for a diversity of housing forms, increased densities and land use and public transport integration, including a shift away from private-car dependency. The emergence of a more compact city aspiration was accompanied by the rise of a neo-liberal approach to governance (explained below), instigating a shift to market-driven flexibility in the planning system. Development approvals were expedited at the demands of powerful development and construction industries. Yet the majority of the Australian community remained unconvinced of the appeals of higher-density living—and the approach escape critical review by Australian researchers (see, for example, Troy 1996). While consolidation was promoted as a government planning strategy, market demand and subsequent housing provision continued to be low-density and dispersed.

Throughout the 1990s and into the 21st Century, the popularity of the detached dwelling and life in relatively isolated suburbs has continued to be challenged, primarily by planning policy and property developers (Searle 2007). Higher-density urban living has also been supported by some demographic groups, including the younger generation, who have been inspired to start their housing careers with the purchase of a more affordable apartment. Urban containment through consolidation has remained the desired metropolitan planning outcome in most cities. Reflecting one of the key rationales for densification is reduced private-car dependence. Accordingly, the provision of public transport around higher-density areas has, for the most part, become a priority. Much of this density is in inner urban areas close to central business districts. However, at the time of writing in 2019, higher-density infill developments are increasingly commonplace in middle ring suburbs, although density in the outer suburban reaches remains relatively low. New construction in these areas is characterised by detached houses rather than townhouses or apartment buildings. Often this is justified by both the planning system and the development industry on the basis of improving housing affordability and satisfying a perceived market demand for privacy and space over apartment living. As a result, in many Australian cities, housing continues to push into isolated and car-dependent outskirts in a relatively uncoordinated way. By global standards, Australian cities remain characterised by urban sprawl and dependent on the private car for transport. This backdrop—private car reliance and continued urban sprawl—provides unique challenges for the development of healthy built environments in Australia.

Australia's Governance

In the introduction to this book, we described Australia's shameful legacy of ill-treatment of its Indigenous peoples. This invasion started officially on 26 January 1788, when a fleet of nine tall ships carrying approximately

650 convicts landed at Botany Bay (now known as Sydney) and went on to claim the continent as a penal colony of the British Empire. It was not until over 100 years later, on 1 January 1901, that Australia was declared an independent nation under a single constitution. Today, Australia remains a constitutional monarchy—'constitutional' because the powers of the Australian government are defined by its own written constitution and 'monarchy' because Australia's Head of State is Her Majesty Queen Elizabeth II.

Contemporary Australian government follows the British (Westminster) tradition. The Governor-General, representing the Crown, exercises the supreme executive power of the Commonwealth. In reality, the head of the Commonwealth government, the Prime Minister, advises the Governor-General, who then acts accordingly. The Prime Minister and the cabinet of ministers he or she leads are appointed by the Governor-General on the advice of the political party that represents a majority of the House of Representatives in the Federal Parliament.

Power is divided between the Commonwealth (also referred to as Federal) government and six State governments. As noted previously, there are also two Territories comprising the mainland of Australia. Each State has its own State constitution and is permitted to pass laws related to any matter not controlled by the Commonwealth under Section 51 of the Australian Constitution. This includes matters relating to health, the environment (including urban planning), education, law enforcement and infrastructure. In addition, across the country are more than 560 Local government authorities known generally as Local Councils. Although these local authorities play a substantial role in the governance of urban planning in Australia, and are arguably the scale of government closest to the people, it is often Commonwealth and State authority that prevails over Local government preferences. At all scales of government in Australia are representatives elected democratically via popular voting, which is compulsory.

The following sections provide a brief outline of the governance of land use planning and health in Australia. We introduce some of the ways different scales of government have embraced (or otherwise) health as an urban planning concern. We emphasise that our review is brief. For more detail on the planning system in Australia, we recommend the texts *Australian urban land use planning: Principles, systems and practice* by Nicole Gurran (2011) and *Planning Australia: An Overview of Urban and Regional Planning*, edited by Susan Thompson with Paul Maginn (2012). For more detail on the operation of the health system in Australia, we recommend the Australian Institute of Health and Welfare's biennial reports on the nation's health, the most recent being *Australia's Health 2018* (Australian Institute of Health and Welfare 2018).

The Governance of Land Use Planning in Australia

Commonwealth Government

Australia's planning system is distributed across the three levels of government described above: Commonwealth, State and Local. Commonwealth involvement in urban decision-making is limited, reflecting the constitutional division of powers. There are, however, several ways that the Commonwealth government can, and does, influence land use planning in Australia. At the time of writing, Commonwealth involvement in cities is channelled through the *Smart Cities Plan*, released in 2016. The plan supports several concepts relevant to healthy planning. For example, it acknowledges the importance of green space and promotes active transport. The key operational mechanism for this plan is through 'City Deals'. These are formal collaborations between all scales of government as well as private-industry partners. They focus on particular sites around the nation deemed to be transitional and with the potential to generate nationwide economic and social impact. While these 'deals' are a welcome channel for Federal interest and funding, this scale of government commitment to urban affairs is constantly shifting, resulting in some scepticism among professions and communities.

State Governments

State government is the key scale of governance in Australia responsible for governing land use. As a result, there are eight different planning systems across Australia's States and Territories. In each, the system is guided by overarching statutory (legislative) planning instruments that regulate development. As well, every State maintains a strategic planning program intended to guide future planning outcomes. Strategic plans are generally not legislated, although their consideration in development assessment may be. Indeed, the historical aim of strategic planning in general is to guide the process of agenda-setting and community collaboration, rather than articulate hard targets for land use management (Albrechts et al. 2016).

It is only quite recently that we have seen these State land use planning systems start to assume some responsibility for health as a planning issue. Starting from the very pinnacle of each State's planning system, some State governments are now including different interpretations of health concepts in the legislatively articulated 'Objectives' (also referred to as 'Objects') of their planning systems. Objectives are extremely significant in that they articulate how planning legislation is to be interpreted. Indeed, any land use decision made contrary to an Act's objective can be deemed unlawful (Gurran 2011). Inclusion of the promotion of health and wellbeing as an objective of planning legislation is therefore a powerful tool for promoting consideration of human health in urban planning decisions. To date, three Australian States have made reference to health or wellbeing in their Objectives (see Table 1.2). While most other States reference related concepts (such as amenity and sustainability), we believe inclusion of the actual word 'health' in primary legislation is an important component of any progression towards having health formally recognised as an urban planning consideration in Australia.

Table 1.3 Summary of the inclusion of health concepts in Australia's primary planning legislation

Jurisdiction	Primary planning legislation	References to healthy built environment concepts in objectives
Commonwealth	Environment Protection and Biodiversity Conservation Act 1999	No
New South Wales	Environmental Planning and Assessment Act 1979	Inserted 2017: 'to promote the proper construction and maintenance of buildings, including the protection of the health and safety of their occupants'
Victoria	Planning and Environment Act 1987	No
Queensland	Planning Act 2016	Inserted 2016: 'to maintain the cultural, economic, physical and social wellbeing of people and communities'.
Western Australia	Planning and Development Act 2005	No
South Australia	Planning, Development and Infrastructure Act 2016	No
Tasmania	Land Use Planning and Approvals Act 1993	Inserted 2015: 'to promote the health and wellbeing of all Tasmanians and visitors to Tasmania by ensuring a pleasant, efficient and safe environment for working, living and recreation'
Northern Territory	Planning Act 2003	No
Australian Capital Territory	Australian Capital Territory (Planning and Land Management) Act 1988 Planning and Development Act 2007	No

In addition to statutory planning instruments, most States also maintain a strategic direction, which is usually articulated in a strategic plan for both its major metropolitan capital and regions. These plans are constantly shifting to accommodate both political intentions and the mood of the jurisdiction (Searle and Bunker 2010). Again, it is now quite common to see health and health-related concepts included as key considerations in these plans. Most State strategic plans—particularly those for large city regions—make reference to liveability, if not health and wellbeing more directly, as a key intention. Once more, we advocate that to ensure health is considered seriously as a planning matter across the Australian States, these plans need to actually use the term 'health' as well as clearly articulate an understanding of what it means to support a healthy built environment.

Local Councils

Each State government delegates different planning responsibilities to Local Councils, such as local development approvals, some infrastructure provisions and local service delivery. Local Councils are a creation of the States, generally deriving their powers solely from State legislation. As a result, State governments can amend the roles and functions of Local government at any time. In reality, State governments are constantly making 'improvements' to Local government, particularly to their land use planning processes. These tend to be characterised by centralisation. They include Local government amalgamations, appointment of planning administrators and planning decision-making panels and the 'calling-in' of (otherwise Local) planning and development decisions by State planning ministers on the grounds of 'State significance'.

Our recent experiences working with Local government in Australia suggest that health, as a planning concern, finds a receptive and enthusiastic audience with planning professionals at this level. Australian research, however, suggests that this professional interest is frequently checked by the politics of Local government (McCosker et al. 2018).

The Governance of Health in Australia

Similar to urban planning, health is a portfolio managed primarily at the scale of the State in Australia. As a result, each State has developed a unique health system over time as a way to administer the vast responsibilities and costs of maintaining a healthy population. Often this reflects a combination of principles, pragmatic politics and historical legacy, rather than the most effective approach to the care of the population.

The Commonwealth government defines overall expectations for health and allocates funding to States for public sector health services.

The Commonwealth also directly subsidises costs associated with primary healthcare services. State governments assume practical responsibility for the provision of public health services, including hospitals. Local governments have responsibility for a somewhat random collection of health functions, such as monitoring food safety in shops and restaurants and providing sanitation services. Adding to the complexity of the health system in Australia is the fact that it is a dual system, comprising public and private sectors. All Australians have affordable access to the healthcare services and medicines deemed necessary for the appropriate treatment of a patient. However, those willing and able to pay can access additional services provided by the private health industry.

The design of this three-tiered healthcare system, defined concurrently by both public and private interests, has several implications for the health of Australians. While healthcare in Australia is of a very high standard, health is an incredibly expensive portfolio, and the health budget is finite. The fundamental aim of the health system is, therefore, to provide a high level of healthcare from a limited resource base. Politicians at the National and State level are charged with making decisions on what the health system should and should not fund. This exposes the provision of health services to social, political and economic pressures, which inevitably influence the way funding is provided and used. As a result, health priorities are often fiercely debated. It is in this adversarial environment that decisions to support initiatives that have an immediate outcome are able to prevail over funding for more 'slow-burning' preventive measures, such as those required by healthy built environments.

In the introduction to this book, we outlined the ideological space in which the notion of healthy planning in Australia has found a home. Planning built environments that support health is what many Australian planners know as best-practice urban planning (Allender et al. 2009). And the elements of social life affected by planning are those health professionals known as the social determinants of health. The challenge today remains in navigating action on this ideological space through existing and ingrained approaches to research, policy and governance. This challenge is known as healthy planning. It has become the subject of a burgeoning amount of research, scholarship and education in Australia, some of which has filtered through to policy, including legislation (Table 1.2). In Figure 1.3, we present a conceptual timeline of selected key moments in the emergent and growing field of healthy planning in Australia. We have included policies, programs, research, education initiatives and particular events (admittedly filtered through our knowledge and involvement). Rather than a comprehensive history, the timeline is intended to provide a sense of the ebb and flow of involvement and multisectoral interest in the emerging field of healthy planning across Australia.

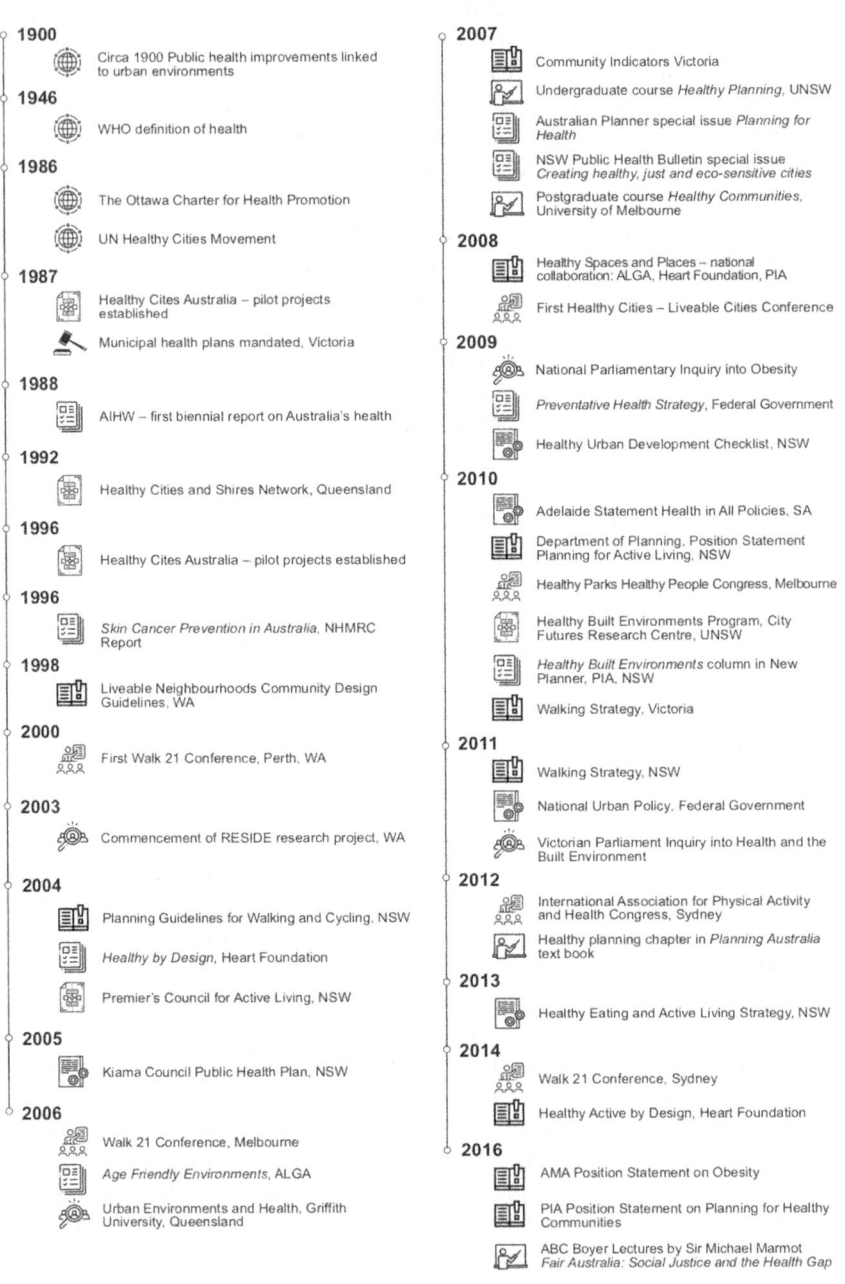

1900
Circa 1900 Public health improvements linked to urban environments

1946
WHO definition of health

1986
The Ottawa Charter for Health Promotion

UN Healthy Cities Movement

1987
Healthy Cites Australia – pilot projects established

Municipal health plans mandated, Victoria

1988
AIHW – first biennial report on Australia's health

1992
Healthy Cities and Shires Network, Queensland

1996
Healthy Cites Australia – pilot projects established

1996
Skin Cancer Prevention in Australia, NHMRC Report

1998
Liveable Neighbourhoods Community Design Guidelines, WA

2000
First Walk 21 Conference, Perth, WA

2003
Commencement of RESIDE research project, WA

2004
Planning Guidelines for Walking and Cycling, NSW

Healthy by Design, Heart Foundation

Premier's Council for Active Living, NSW

2005
Kiama Council Public Health Plan, NSW

2006
Walk 21 Conference, Melbourne

Age Friendly Environments, ALGA

Urban Environments and Health, Griffith University, Queensland

2007
Community Indicators Victoria

Undergraduate course Healthy Planning, UNSW

Australian Planner special issue Planning for Health

NSW Public Health Bulletin special issue Creating healthy, just and eco-sensitive cities

Postgraduate course Healthy Communities, University of Melbourne

2008
Healthy Spaces and Places – national collaboration: ALGA, Heart Foundation, PIA

First Healthy Cities – Liveable Cities Conference

2009
National Parliamentary Inquiry into Obesity

Preventative Health Strategy, Federal Government

Healthy Urban Development Checklist, NSW

2010
Adelaide Statement Health in All Policies, SA

Department of Planning, Position Statement Planning for Active Living, NSW

Healthy Parks Healthy People Congress, Melbourne

Healthy Built Environments Program, City Futures Research Centre, UNSW

Healthy Built Environments column in New Planner, PIA, NSW

Walking Strategy, Victoria

2011
Walking Strategy, NSW

National Urban Policy, Federal Government

Victorian Parliament Inquiry into Health and the Built Environment

2012
International Association for Physical Activity and Health Congress, Sydney

Healthy planning chapter in Planning Australia text book

2013
Healthy Eating and Active Living Strategy, NSW

2014
Walk 21 Conference, Sydney

Healthy Active by Design, Heart Foundation

2016
AMA Position Statement on Obesity

PIA Position Statement on Planning for Healthy Communities

ABC Boyer Lectures by Sir Michael Marmot Fair Australia: Social Justice and the Health Gap

Figure 1.3 Key events in healthy planning in Australia

Conclusion: The Ethos of Governance in Australia

Having explained the basic characteristics of our people and urban areas, as well as described the structure and systems of governance that underpin our approach to urban planning and health, we conclude with some reflections on the general ethos, or philosophy, underpinning decision-making in this country.

It was not long after Australia was settled as a British colony that the concept of a 'fair go' emerged as central to Australian life. Although by no means without conflict, the colony's relative isolation from the motherland of Britain, combined with the harsh biophysical environment, bound new communities around a collective trade-off of a hard life with the equal access to opportunities to 'get ahead'. This was a relatively new notion for many people coming from Britain, where the class system was rife and social mobility a rarity.

The 'fair go' concept remains important in discourse on governance in Australia. This belief in access to opportunity, however, should not be confused with the idea that Australia is a nation aspiring to intrinsic equality. Opportunity in Australia has always been contingent on hard work and aspiration. Prospects for advancement have been posited as available to all, but progress has realistically been within the reach of only those able to put in the effort. During periods of prosperity, Australian governments have used the 'fair go' mantra to maintain a relatively interventionist approach, seeking to remove disadvantage and implement safety nets for those unable to take advantage of opportunities. More recently, however, the Australian notion of a 'fair go' has been co-opted. It is now used to justify policies of deregulation, where opportunity is increasingly provisional on competition, personal and professional connections and chance.

This embrace of deregulation was initiated during the 1980s as a direct response to global trends. Australian political discourse followed other countries, particularly the United Kingdom, to position the government as a competitive, market-driven entity, rather than a public provider. Since that time, a range of structural and cultural changes have worked their way through Australian governance. They are widely recognised as a trend towards 'neo-liberalism'. This is a term used to refer to a system of governance in which the free market is empowered. Neo-liberalism is generally associated with policies such as cutting trade tariffs and barriers, selling off public assets, limiting the power of trade unions, lowering company and personal taxation and the privatisation of public service provision (including health). These policy reforms were rolled out throughout the end of the 20th Century to deregulate the Australian economy, passing key decision-making processes over to the invisible, yet persuasive, 'hand of the market' (Smith 1776).

There are many different views of neo-liberalism. These cover not just its political origins but also its ethical implications. We are by no means advocating that a neo-liberal approach should be completely abandoned by the Australian governance ethos. Based on our knowledge and experience as urban planners, however, we do urge awareness and, where required, temperance of the market as a decision-maker. It is our hope that this book demonstrates that, if anything, healthy built environments in Australia require ongoing checks to market-based urban planning systems.

The next chapter reviews some of the key health issues and opportunities in Australia. Our key message is that good health in this country must remain relatively accessible to all. Providing health-supportive built environments is an effective and imperative component of health equity in this country.

References

Albrechts, l., Balducci, A. and Hillier Abingdon, J. (2016) *Situated Practices of Strategic Planning: An International Perspective*, Routledge, New York.

Alexander, S. (2017) *Australia's changing age structure–Is it all just about ageing?*.id The Population Experts, Melbourne, https://blog.id.com.au/ [Accessed 26 July 2018].

Allender, S., Gleeson, E., Crammond, B., Sacks, G., Lawrence, M., Peeters, A., Loff, B. and Swinburn, B. (2009) Moving beyond 'rates, roads and rubbish': How do local governments make choices about healthy public policy to prevent obesity? *Australia and New Zealand Health Policy*, 6(1) p. 20.

Australian Bureau of Statistics (2017) *Australian Demographic Statistics, June 2017*, Cat. no. 3101.0, Australian Bureau of Statistics, Canberra.

Australian Institute of Health and Welfare (2018) *Australia's Health 2018*, Australian Institute of Health and Welfare, Canberra.

Deacon, M. (2016) *Three Growth Markets in Australia: A Demographic Analysis*.id The Population Experts, Melbourne, https://blog.id.com.au [Accessed 26 July 2018].

Gurran, N. (2011) *Australian Urban Land Use Planning: Principles, Systems and Practice*, 2nd edition, Sydney University Press, Sydney, NSW.

Forster, C. (2006) The challenge of change: Australian cities and Urban planning in the new millennium. *Geographical Research*, 44(2) pp. 173–182.

Hamnett, S. and Freestone, R. (2000) *The Australian Metropolis: A Planning History*, Allen & Unwin, Sydney, NSW.

Leigh, A. (2013) *Battlers and Billionaires: The Story of Inequality in Australia*, Black Inc Books, Melbourne.

McCosker, A., Matan, A. and Marinova, D. (2018) Policies, politics, and paradigms: Healthy planning in Australian local government. *Sustainability*, 10(4) p. 1008.

OECD (2018) Income inequality (indicator). doi:10.1787/459aa7f1-en, https://www.oecd-ilibrary.org/social-issues-migration-health/income-inequality/indicator/english_459aa7f1-en [Accessed 26 July 2018].

Searle, G. (2007) *Sydney's Urban Consolidation Experience: Power, Politics and Community*, Research Paper 12, Urban Research Program, Griffith University, Brisbane.

Searle, G. and Bunker, R. (2010) Metropolitan strategic planning: An Australian paradigm? *Planning Theory*, 9(3) pp. 163–180.

Smith, A. (1776) *An Inquiry into the Nature and Causes of the Wealth of Nations*, ed. Rees-Mogg, W. (1995), Taylor and Francis, London.

Thompson, S. M. and Maginn, P. eds. (2012) *Planning Australia*, 2nd edition, Cambridge University Press, Melbourne.

Troy, P. (1996) *The Perils of Urban Consolidation*, Federation Press, Sydney, NSW.

2 Australia's Health

Introduction

What do we mean when we say a person is 'healthy'? In the introduction to this book, we cited the widely accepted view of the World Health Organization (WHO) to propose that health is much more than the presence or absence of disease. Instead, it is a complete state of mental, social and physical wellbeing (WHO 1948). In this book, we explicitly promote the notion that health in Australia is about so much more than simply preventing death or extending life expectancy. It must also be about quality of life and the ability to contribute to the rich fabric of a sustainable society.

Obviously, there are degrees of good and bad health, and these change over a person's lifetime. Health is shaped by an individual's genetic inheritance and past and present lifestyle. It also reflects their experiences of socio-economic, cultural and physical environments, which include access to health infrastructure over the life course. Such infrastructure comprises hospitals and general practitioners but also extends to the green open spaces, cycleways and community facilities that make up healthy built environments.

When seeking to actualise better health, a person's health can be conceptualised as dependent on two factors: 'determinants' (baseline things that influence health) and 'interventions' (things that can be done to protect and improve a person's health). In terms of determinants, we are particularly interested in the impact of what is known as the social determinants of health (Wilkinson and Marmot 2003). These are differentiated from more natural and obvious determinants of health, such as a person's genetic or biophysical make-up. Social determinants of health arise from structures, processes and conditions that are socially created, and they are inextricably related to the way we organise society. They are the social, economic, political, cultural and environmental 'conditions into which people are born, grow, live, work and age' (WHO 2018). Throughout this book, we demonstrate the way many of Australia's most destructive and expensive health problems have their origins in social determinants and associated inequalities.

In terms of interventions, we are especially interested in the multiple ways built environments can be modified and managed to promote health and prevent illness. Contemporary health systems, including those in Australia, often focus on treating people once they are sick, rather than concentrating on the things that are making them unwell in the first place. A more progressive model will seek to intervene and change aspects of the environment that contribute to ill health, rather than simply deal with illness after it appears or blame the individual for their response to the environment around them.

The remainder of this chapter looks at Australia's health from a number of angles. We examine the burden of disease in the Australian population and the important role of prevention. Inequality in exposure to health risks and, by implication, health outcomes is an important and recurrent theme. In this chapter, we demonstrate the way people living in rural and remote areas, people living with the lowest socio-economic status and Aboriginal and Torres Strait Islander people fare worse than others in terms of their health and longevity. We conclude with a brief introduction to some of the key risk factors facing modern Australia.

Are Australians 'Healthy'?

According to many indicators, Australia enjoys good health relative to populations of comparable countries within the Organization for Economic Co-operation and Development (OECD) (see Figure 2.1). Life expectancy at birth, commonly used to assess the overall health of a population, has climbed steadily over time and is now more than 30 years longer than it was in the late 1800s. Life expectancy for a boy born in 2016 was 80.4 years, and for a girl, 84.6 years (Australian Institute of Health and Welfare [AIHW] 2018).

While Australians enjoy relatively good health, there are several concerning trends. Non-communicable diseases are increasing across most countries in the world, and Australia is no exception. The term 'non-communicable diseases' literally means diseases one cannot catch from another person. These are also referred to as 'chronic', which simply means diseases that affect a person over a long period, usually at least more than three months. In 2016, the top five leading causes of death in Australia could all be considered non-communicable diseases. They were:

1. Coronary heart disease
2. Dementia and Alzheimer's disease

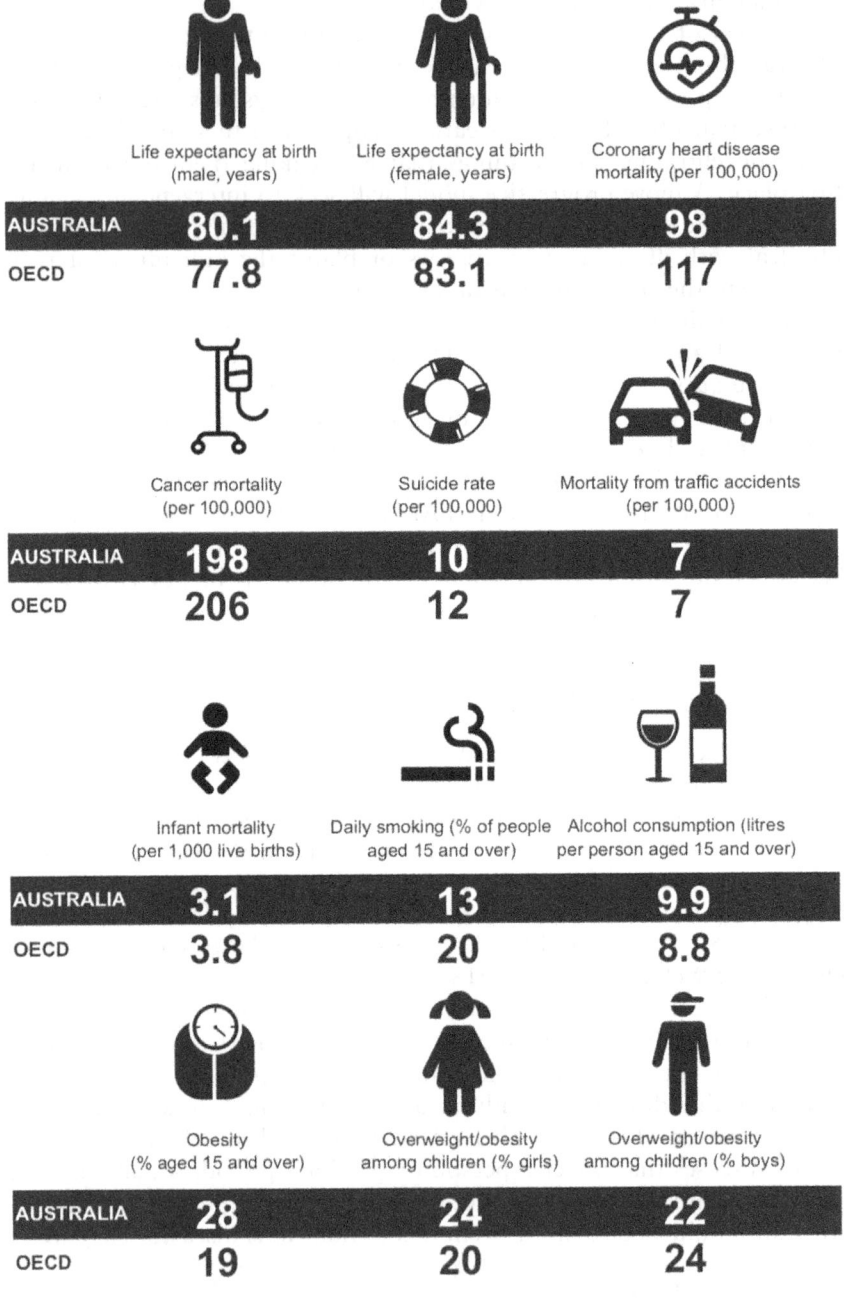

Figure 2.1 Indicators of Australia's health compared with OECD countries

Source: OECD 2014

3. Cerebrovascular disease (for example, stroke)
4. Lung cancer
5. Chronic obstructive pulmonary disease (a group of lung diseases)

(AIHW 2016a)

The scale of the impact from non-communicable diseases has escalated immensely throughout the past 50 years. Much of this increase is related to social and lifestyle changes. For example, until relatively recently, people were more physically active and ate less processed foods. They prepared food at home more often, walked more for transport, and their jobs and day-to-day living involved more physical effort. These practices have now been replaced with convenience eating, private cars for transport, computer-automated manufacturing and labour-saving devices around the home. Modern life is increasingly characterised by the avoidance of movement, also known as sedentary behaviour. We discuss this as a risk factor in Chapter 4—Planning for Physical Activity.

The contemporary dominance of non-communicable diseases in statistics on the causes of death in Australia has several specific features. Firstly, heart disease remains the leading cause of mortality for males and the second most common cause of death for females. Deaths from heart disease have decreased over the past 20 years but still accounted for 13% of male deaths and 11% of female deaths in 2016 (AIHW 2018).

Secondly, the number of new cancer cases diagnosed is increasing in Australia. Diagnosis of cancer more than doubled between 1982 and 2016—from 47,400 to 130,500. This increase can be explained, in part, by the ageing and increasing size of the population and by improvements in the technologies and techniques used to identify and diagnose cancer. Again, other explanations generally implicate behaviours characteristic of modern life, including sedentary behaviour, smoking and unhealthy eating. Of note is that skin cancer is a particularly serious problem in Australia. However, it contributes more to the burden of disease, rather than death, as discussed below.

Thirdly, a relatively new and increasingly problematic trend in Australia is the noticeable rise in deaths from Alzheimer's disease and other dementias. There were close to 12,000 deaths from dementia in 2014 compared with 8200 deaths in 2009. More likely to affect women, dementia became Australia's second leading cause of death in 2013, surpassing strokes. Much of this can be explained by the fact that the population is ageing, suggesting it is not a cause that is likely to retract in the near future.

A final note on causes of death in Australia is that while non-communicable diseases account for the vast majority of mortality and morbidity in this nation, different age and population groups have vastly different leading causes of death. For example, in 2016, transport accidents were the leading underlying cause of death among people aged 1–14, comprising 14% of all deaths. Suicide was the leading underlying cause of death among people aged 15–44, occurring at a rate of 12 deaths per 100,000 people in 2014.

So far, we have focused this discussion on causes of death. The concept of what it means to be 'healthy', however, encompasses not just how many years a person lives and how they die but whether those years are lived with disability, chronic illness or other health conditions that affect quality of life. For example, compared with having a life expectancy of 80.4 years, a boy born in 2012 in Australia could expect to live only 62.4 of these years without disability (AIHW 2016a). A burden of disease analysis can be used to account for this impact. This technique quantifies fatal (for example, death from dementia) and non-fatal (for example, living with dementia) effects of diseases in a consistent manner. These are then combined into a summary measure of health called a disability-adjusted life year, or DALY. The DALY measure combines estimates of years of life lost due to premature death and years lived in ill health or with disability to count the total years of healthy life lost to disease (AIHW 2018).

The most recent burden of disease figures for Australia are from 2011 and were published by the Australian Institute of Health and Welfare in 2016 (AIHW 2016b). At this time, there were 201 years of life lost due to premature death or living with disease or injury for every 1,000 people in Australia—equivalent to 4.5 million DALYs. This burden was distributed almost evenly between burden from dying early and burden due to living with disease or injury. It is positive to note that this is a decrease of 10% from 2003. The health issues that caused the greatest burden in 2011 were cancer, cardiovascular diseases, mental illnesses, substance use disorders, musculoskeletal conditions and injuries. At the disease level, coronary heart disease, lung cancer, other musculoskeletal conditions, back pain and problems, chronic obstructive pulmonary disease and lung cancer caused the most burden.

The remainder of this chapter reviews some of the inequalities facing Australia today and concludes with an introduction to risk factors for ill health. For a more rigorous and comprehensive exploration of Australia's health, we urge readers to access the AHIW's biennial reports on the nation's health, the most recent being *Australia's Health 2018* (AIHW 2018).

Inequalities in Health

To this point, we have presented a broad picture of Australia's health status, which is a relatively positive portrayal. Unfortunately, these general figures mask some substantial pockets of inequality. Of particular concern is the relatively poor health of people living outside our major cities, the stark socio-economic gradient to many health outcomes across the nation and the ongoing gap between the health of the Aboriginal and Torres Strait Islander people and the nation as a whole.

Health in Regional and Remote Australia

In Chapter 1—Australia and Australia's Planning—we introduced Australia as a nation of urban dwellers. In 2016, over 67% of the population lived in one of the country's eight largest cities. This leaves 33% of the population distributed throughout the remainder of our large continent (Australian Bureau of Statistics 2017). In very general terms, this third of the population have poorer health.

Analysing the differences in health and welfare of non-city inhabitants depends on the ability to classify areas according to their remoteness. Over the last 20 years, a number of geographical classifications for Australia have emerged. The AIHW recommends the use of the *Australian Statistical Geography Standard Remoteness Areas* classification. This unique classification allocates areas of land to one of five categories based on the distance people have to travel by road to access centres of various sizes:

1. Major cities
2. Inner regional
3. Outer regional
4. Remote Australia
5. Very remote Australia

Because of small population sizes, data for outer regional, remote and very remote areas are often combined for reporting purposes and referred to as simply remote. We follow this protocol.

Table 2.1 Behaviour risk factors by remoteness in Australia

Remoteness	Major cities	Inner regional	Outer regional and remote
% of total population	71%	18%	11%
Behavioural risk factors (age standardised prevalence ratio)			
Tobacco smoking	1.00	1.15	1.30
Harmful alcohol consumption	1.00	1.16	1.30
Lack of physical activity	1.00	1.09	1.24
Consuming recommended intake of fruit	1.00	0.98	0.90
Consuming recommended intake of vegetables	1.00	1.44	1.54

Source: AIHW 2016a

Table 2.1 presents data on the prevalence of several key behavioural risk factors by remoteness. While fewer than three in 10 people (29%) live in regional and remote areas, deaths in these areas accounted for almost two in five (38%) of the premature deaths occurring in Australia in 2011–2013. People in regional and remote areas were more likely to have arthritis, asthma, heart disease and a number of other chronic health conditions (AIHW 2016a). People living in regional and remote areas were also, on average, more likely than their urban counterparts to engage in unhealthy lifestyle behaviours, such as smoking, insufficient physical activity and risky alcohol consumption. These gradients generally follow the degree of remoteness. For example, in 2016, the premature mortality rate among people living in remote areas was 1.6 times as high as the rate among people in major cities. In very remote areas, it was 2.2 times as high (AIHW 2016a).

A range of social, demographic, cultural and environmental factors underpin this distinctly geographical expression of health and wellness across Australia. This book focuses on Australia's urban environments, and as such, it is beyond its remit to examine the incredibly complex pathways that place the health of rural and regional Australians below the national average. For interested readers, we encourage exploration of the work of the National Rural Health Alliance. In general, while reduced access to educational and employment opportunities and lower incomes are undoubtedly contributing factors to the urban rural health gap, a deficit in the availability of health professionals in rural areas may also be a contributing factor (National Rural Health Alliance 2016).

Socio-Economic Groups

> Disadvantage has many forms and may be absolute or relative. It can include having few family assets, having a poorer education during adolescence, having insecure employment, becoming stuck in a hazardous or dead-end job, living in poor housing, trying to bring up a family in difficult circumstances and living on an inadequate retirement pension. These disadvantages tend to concentrate among the same people, and their effects on health accumulate during life. The longer people live in stressful economic and social circumstances, the greater the physiological wear and tear they suffer, and the less likely they are to enjoy a healthy old age.
>
> (Wilkinson and Marmot 2003, p. 10)

The quote above is from a landmark report commissioned by the WHO: *Social determinants of health—the solid facts*. The report remains an insightful source of information on the complex links between wealth and health that characterise the distribution of illness across the world today.

Similar to the geographical distribution described above, inequalities in health also appear in the form of a social gradient. In general, the higher a person's socio-economic position in a society, the healthier they are. This is because health outcomes are sensitive to surrounding social conditions. Factors such as income, education, employment, empowerment and social support act to strengthen or undermine health and wellbeing. These are the social determinants of health—the 'causes of the causes'—or underlying factors that influence other health determinants. Understanding this concept is vital to the pursuit of healthy built environments.

The WHO defines the social determinants of health as the conditions in which people are born, grow, live, work and age (WHO 2018). These circumstances are shaped by the distribution of money, power and resources at global, national and local levels. The fact that these things influence health is demonstrated by persistent evidence that people from diminished social or economic circumstances are at greater risk of poor health, have higher rates of illness, disability and death and live shorter lives than those who are more advantaged. Generally, every step up the socio-economic ladder is accompanied by an increase in health.

Table 2.2 demonstrates that this gradient is alive and well in modern Australia. It presents several key risk factors for some of Australia's most prevalent chronic diseases. For example, people in the lowest socio-economic group are more likely to smoke, more likely to be overweight or obese and less likely to engage in sufficient physical activity—some of the key behavioural risk factors for the common chronic diseases across the country.

There are several explanations for the social gradient of health in Australia. Like so many of the concepts explored in this book, its presence and influence reflect a complex confluence of structures and social practices, which are reinforced by prevailing political, economic and cultural ideologies. Occupation is often cited as a contributing factor. Although

Table 2.2 Risk factors for chronic disease by socio-economic status

Risk factors	Lowest quintile of socio-economic groups (%)	Highest quintile of socio-economic groups (%)
Low birthweight	7.5	5.6
Daily smoking	20	6.7
Inactive or insufficiently active	76	56
Overweight or obese	66	58
High blood pressure	26	21

Source: AIHW 2016a

Australia regularly claims to be an egalitarian nation, a person's job, including whether or not they are employed, still shapes their position in society. Employment in higher-status occupations is commonly associated with higher education levels. Education promotes resilience, enabling people to make informed decisions about things that affect their health. Besides improving socio-economic position, a better job is usually accompanied by a higher income, which allows for greater access to goods and services that provide health benefits, such as better food and housing, additional healthcare options and greater capacity to make healthy choices about behaviours such as physical activity and dietary intake. Related to the discussion above on regional and remote Australia, the sheer distances that separate some Australians also, inevitably, play a part. In Chapter 1—Australia and Australia's Planning—we demonstrated the way that socio-economic status has a geographical expression across our nation, with areas of disadvantage overwhelmingly concentrated in rural and regional areas. This is where it is most difficult to provide continuity of health services, from education on prevention to actual health treatment.

One of the world's most respected authorities on the concept of health equity is Sir Michael Marmot. Sir Marmot, born in the United Kingdom and educated at the University of Sydney, has pioneered conceptualisations and awareness of health equity around the world through his work on the social determinants of health. In 2016, he addressed health equity in Australia through a series of recordings for the publicly acclaimed series known as the 'Boyer Lectures'. Transcripts of the presentation have subsequently been published (Marmot 2016), and we recommend them to readers interested in the socio-economic gradient to health in Australia.

Aboriginal and Torres Strait Islander People

This book opened with acknowledgement of the Aboriginal and Torres Strait Islander people as the custodians of the Australian land. This is a culture that goes back at least 60,000 years, adapting over this time to live in harmony with the Australian environment. It was destroyed, rapidly and violently, from the very first moment of the British invasion in 1788. The following excerpt of a report by journalist Edward Wilson is telling:

> In less than twenty years we have nearly swept them off the face of the earth. We have shot them down like dogs. In the guise of friendship we have issued corrosive sublimate in their damper and consigned whole tribes to the agonies of an excruciating death. We have made them drunkards, and infected them with diseases which have

rotted the bones of their adults, and made such few children as are born amongst them a sorrow and a torture from the very instant of their birth. We have made them outcasts on their own land, and are rapidly consigning them to entire annihilation.

Edward Wilson, The Argus, 17 March 1856
(in Harris 2013, pp. 5–6)

Wilson was writing from Melbourne (settled in the 1830s), yet the rapid devastation of the indigenous population that accompanied the Europeans was shockingly commonplace. Sadly, the legacy of ill-treatment and poor health described above has continued through the 20th Century. Now, almost 20 years into the 21st Century, the Aboriginal and Torres Strait Islander people continue to experience poor health outcomes relative to the rest of the nation.

Strikingly, this inequality is pervasive to the very core of the culture, starting with intrinsic evaluations of health. Aboriginal and Torres Strait Islander people rate their own general health as poorer than that of other Australians. The differences between the two populations' perceptions are great, which is consistent with other measures of overall health status. In 2010–2012, compared with non-Indigenous Australians, life expectancy for Aboriginal and Torres Strait Islander people was estimated to be 10.6 years lower for males (69.1 compared with 79.7 years) and 9.5 years lower for females (73.7 compared with 83.1 years) (AIHW 2016a). In 2012, most (70%) Aboriginal and Torres Strait Islander adults reported low/moderate levels of psychological stress, and 30% had high/very high levels. After adjusting for differences in the age structure of the two populations, the Indigenous Australian rate of high/very high psychological distress was 2.7 times the rate for non-Aboriginal and Torres Strait Islander adults. Related to this is the suicide rate for Aboriginal and Torres Strait Islander people, which sits at approximately twice the rate compared with non-Indigenous Australians. Among Aboriginal and Torres Strait Islander people aged 15–19, the suicide rate is five times the non-Indigenous rate (AIHW 2016a).

The health disparities between Aboriginal and Torres Strait Islander people and non-Indigenous populations are not geographically even, with communities in remote and rural areas and the Northern Territory generally reporting lower health status and outcomes. For example, Indigenous life expectancy is estimated to be lower in the Northern Territory than in any other jurisdiction. Life expectancy for Indigenous males was estimated to be 63.4 years compared with 70.5 years for New South Wales (a gap of 7.1 years) while Indigenous females had a life expectancy estimate of 68.7 years compared with 74.6 years for New South Wales (a gap of 5.9 years).

Implicated in the contemporary disadvantage of many Indigenous people is the legacy of colonisation, which separated Aboriginal and Torres Strait Islander people from their lands and subjected them to state control regarding every aspect of their lives. Low income, the absence of affordable housing, discrimination and cultural differences in connections to home, family, kinship and country are contributing factors (Keys Young 1999). This is compounded by policies of past and present governments that have fostered distrust when it comes to Aboriginal and Torres Strait Islander people engaging with 'white' services, including health services (Habibis 2011).

Risk Factors

Any behaviour or experience that augments vulnerability to ill health or injury is known as a risk factor. Some risk factors are regarded as causes of disease; others are correlated with, or implicated in, ongoing experiences of ill health. Risk factors can be a product of an individual's lifestyle—for example, physical inactivity. They can also be ingrained in the built or social environment in which an individual lives and works—for example, a lack of transport options alternative to the private car. These two examples—physical inactivity and car dependency—demonstrate the way environmental risk factors (car dependency) predispose an individual to lifestyle risk factors (sedentary behaviour). As with most concepts, when it comes to healthy built environments, the impact of risk factors is rarely isolated or simple.

Many of the risk factors implicated in mortality and morbidity in Australia are described as modifiable. This means that their impact could be reduced by individual behaviour changes or changes to the environment around the individual. It is interesting to consider constraints to the concept of modifiability, however. While it may be easy to say that car dependency can be modified by encouraging alternative transport modes, to a road engineer seeking to retrofit a sprawling city designed around the car, this 'ability to modify' is much more complex.

In Part II of this book, we examine four risk factors in depth: an unhealthy planet, physical inactivity, a lack of social interaction and unhealthy eating. There is, however, a diversity of other risk factors contributing to the burden of disease in Australia. Figure 2.2 lists some of these. While the figure provides an understanding of the diversity of risk factors, we caution that this is not an exclusive list, and that the impact of any one risk factor can rarely be considered independently. In particular, the list of environmental factors is especially limited. As we demonstrate through this book, there are many other elements of the environment, including the built environment, that contribute to the burden of disease in Australia.

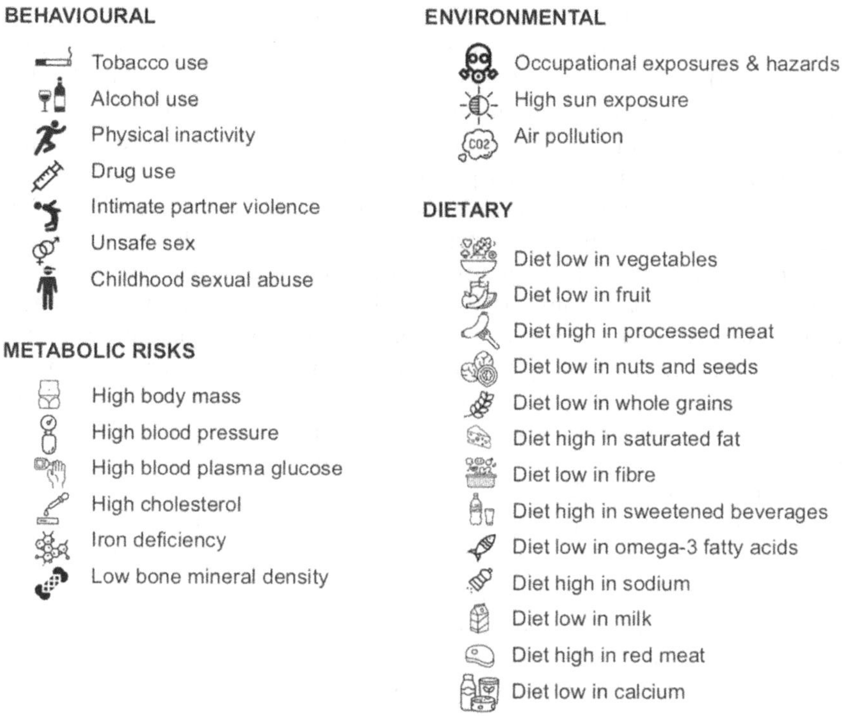

BEHAVIOURAL

- Tobacco use
- Alcohol use
- Physical inactivity
- Drug use
- Intimate partner violence
- Unsafe sex
- Childhood sexual abuse

METABOLIC RISKS

- High body mass
- High blood pressure
- High blood plasma glucose
- High cholesterol
- Iron deficiency
- Low bone mineral density

ENVIRONMENTAL

- Occupational exposures & hazards
- High sun exposure
- Air pollution

DIETARY

- Diet low in vegetables
- Diet low in fruit
- Diet high in processed meat
- Diet low in nuts and seeds
- Diet low in whole grains
- Diet high in saturated fat
- Diet low in fibre
- Diet high in sweetened beverages
- Diet low in omega-3 fatty acids
- Diet high in sodium
- Diet low in milk
- Diet high in red meat
- Diet low in calcium

Figure 2.2 Selected risk factors contributing to the burden of disease in Australia
Source: Adapted from AIHW 2016a

Conclusion

This chapter has painted a picture of Australia as a nation that enjoys relatively good health. In terms of life expectancy, for example, we score well above the international average, and even the average for OECD nations. Against this backdrop, we outlined some of the key diseases that are particularly concerning and costly in Australia. Most of these are long-term (chronic) non-communicable diseases, especially heart disease, dementia and cancer. Many of these diseases have comorbidities with a huge potential to detract from the quality of life of both sufferers and their carers. While these are the most common causes of mortality, they generally impact the older population. There are other worrying trends in the causes of death for younger people, including an escalating suicide rate, deaths from drug overdose and addiction and deaths from accidents, particularly road accidents.

This chapter progressed to examine three of the main sources of inequality in the health of Australians. The gap between the health of rural and urban dwellers is a quintessentially Australian one, with a complex history and geography that must be unravelled if the gap is to narrow. The socio-economic gradient to ill health in this country reflects that of other comparable nations. However, as explored in Chapter 1—Australia and Australia's Planning—of concern is that it is increasing. And finally, the appalling gap between the health of Aboriginal and Torres Strait Islander people and other Australians continues to be a source of shame in a nation as wealthy and prosperous as Australia.

We concluded with a review of some of the risk factors implicated in mortality and morbidity in Australia. Many of these risk factors can be avoided, or at least their impact reduced, by modifications to behaviours, environments and/or combinations of the two. The way the built environment is planned and managed has an integral role to play in this complex dichotomy. This is suggested by the simple fact that changes in the profile of diseases in Australia have occurred concurrent with changes in the way we live in urban areas. The next Part of our book demonstrates that this is also verified with an increasingly robust body of empirical research and knowledge.

This chapter closes the first part of our book, which has introduced Australia, its system of governance and its health. As outlined above, Part II takes four key risk factors that are modifiable through built environment interventions. After describing the nature and extent of each factor in the Australian context, we go on to explore how better planning can decrease their adverse impact on health.

References

Australian Bureau of Statistics (2017) *Australian Demographic Statistics, June 2017*, Cat. no. 3101.0, Australian Bureau of Statistics, Canberra.

Australian Institute of Health and Welfare (2016a) *Australia's Health 2016*, Australian Institute of Health and Welfare, Canberra.

Australian Institute of Health and Welfare (2016b) *Australian Burden of Disease Study: Impact and Causes of Illness and Death in Australia in 2011*. Australian Institute of Health and Welfare, Canberra.

Australian Institute of Health and Welfare (2018) *Australia's Health 2018*, Australian Institute of Health and Welfare, Canberra.

Habibis, D. (2011) A framework for reimagining indigenous mobility and homelessness. *Urban Policy and Research*, 29(4) pp. 401–414.

Keys Young (1999) *Homelessness in the Aboriginal and Torres Strait Islander Context and Its Possible Implications for the Supported Accommodation Assistance Program*, Department of Health and Family Services, Australian Government, Canberra.

Marmot, M. (2016) [radio broadcast] *The 2016 Boyer Lectures–Fair Australia: Social Justice and the Health Gap–Exploring the Challenges Faced by Communities in Solving Issues Around Health Inequality*, ABC Radio National, Melbourne, www.abc.net.au/radionational/programs/boyerlectures/series/2016-boyer-lectures/7802472 [Accessed 26 July 2018].

National Rural Health Alliance (2016) *The Health of People Living in Remote Australia*. National Rural Health Alliance, Deakin West, ACT.

Organization for Economic Co-operation and Development (2014) *How's Life in Your Region? Measuring Regional and Local Well-Being for Policy Making*, Organization for Economic Co-operation and Development Publishing, Paris.

Wilkinson, R. G. and Marmot, M. (2003) *Social Determinants of Health: The Solid Facts*, 2nd edition, World Health Organization, Copenhagen.

Wilson, E. (1856) *Argus*, 17 March 1856, in Harris, J. (2013) *One Blood: 200 Years of Aboriginal Encounter with Christianity: A Story of Hope*, Concilia Ltd, Fullarton, SA.

World Health Organization (1948) *Constitution of the World Health Organization*, World Health Organization, Geneva.

World Health Organization (2018) *Social Determinants of Health*. World Health Organisation, Geneva, www.who.int/social_determinants/sdh_definition/en/ [Accessed 26 July 2018].

Part II

Domains of Wellbeing

Introduction

Part II is comprised of four chapters, each covering a specific 'Domain of Wellbeing'. These Domains focus our review of the ways urban planning can address health in contemporary Australia by looking at each of the following:

- The built environment and planetary health
- The built environment and physical activity
- The built environment and social interaction
- The built environment and healthy eating

While the built environment has the capacity to influence health in many ways, the Domains we propose warrant direct attention for a number of reasons.

Firstly, we take a fresh perspective on the typical risks explored in this space by positioning an unhealthy planet as a risk factor for human health. We start here because, without a healthy planet, ultimately there is no life and pursuit of a healthy built environment is futile. This chapter takes the emergent concept of Planetary Health to present a comprehensive case for urgent action on impending global environmental crises. The following three chapters address the more immediately obvious risk factors for the escalating chronic non-communicable diseases burdening urban populations across the globe. These risk factors are physical inactivity, social isolation and unhealthy eating.

Secondly, the Domains are broad areas where better planning of the built environment has the potential to effect substantial health improvements. And while we focus specifically on Australian health problems, there is wider global applicability. Our Domains are tangible areas where the built environment can most effectively target its support for human health.

Thirdly, the Domains give coherency to a burgeoning base of 'healthy built environment' literature. We have found this relatively simple conceptualisation invaluable in the unpacking and ordering of a vast and increasingly unwieldy body of research in a way that can be readily applied to policy development and areas of evidence paucity. Accordingly, this enhances opportunities for collaboration in the creation of a built environment that supports the health of all communities.

3   Planning for the Health of the Planet

Introduction

We begin the book's second Part—Domains of Wellbeing—with the concept of a healthy planet. We propose that planetary ill health is the most serious risk factor facing human health across the globe. Our survival depends on the planet's life support systems to provide fresh food, clean water, unpolluted air and protection from natural hazards. Without a healthy planet, opportunities to create and maintain a healthy built environment are diminished and ultimately futile.

At the time of writing, Australia faces several unique environmental challenges. Some are a consequence of our nation's fragile geography, harsh climate and vulnerable biodiversity. Most, however, are the result of careless human intervention, including the way Europeans have settled this land, and the resource-intensive practices of living that characterise the Australian way of life.

This chapter first explores the undeniable link between the health of the planet and human health. We then shift to a focus on climate change, which in 2008 was declared a risk to all determinants of health by the World Health Organization. Given the extent of the multiple risks posed to human health, we go on to provide a broad sweep of Australian programs and approaches to climate change. Here, we identify government-, industry-, practitioner- and research-led responses. We also acknowledge the critical role of the Australian community. The chapter concludes by considering how these efforts can be enhanced through greater integration and interconnected thinking, focusing on the notion of co-benefits from action on climate change for human health. This evolving policy initiative provides a positive opportunity for protecting the planet's health as the foundation for developing healthy built environments in Australia.

The Concept of Planetary Health

'Planetary health' is defined as "the health of human civilisations and the natural systems on which they depend" (Lancet Planetary Health 2017, p.e1).

Table 3.1 Status of planetary boundaries

Boundary	Status from human action
Climate change	Transgressed—within increasing risk zone
Ocean acidification	Within safe operating boundary
Stratospheric ozone	Within safe operating boundary
Biogeochemical nitrogen cycle	Transgressed—in high-risk zone
Phosphorus cycle	Transgressed—in high-risk zone
Global freshwater use	Within safe operating boundary
Land system change	Transgressed—within increasing risk zone
Rate of biodiversity loss	Transgressed—in high-risk zone
Chemical pollution	Boundary level not determined
Atmospheric aerosol loading	Boundary level not determined

Source: Adapted from Rockström et al. 2009; Steffen et al. 2015

It is an interdisciplinary and transdisciplinary approach to health that places human beings at the centre of both the impacts and causes of an impending global environmental crisis. This specific model of planetary health is the latest in a legacy of recognition of the dependency of human health on the health of our planet. Barton and Grant's famous Settlement Health Map (Barton and Grant 2006), for example, equates the health of the planet with the global ecosystem, which incorporates biodiversity, resource conservation and climate stability. Another interesting way to conceptualise planetary and human health is the concept of 'planetary boundaries'. These define 'safe limits' for human activity in relation to different and yet highly interrelated 'earth system processes' (Rockström et al. 2009; Steffen et al. 2015). Moving beyond the safe limit of a boundary may result in serious, and possibly catastrophic, environmental consequences, with related immediate and long-term health implications. Table 3.1 shows the identified planetary boundaries and their current status relative to human impact.

The links between planetary and human health are complex and interconnected, as well as contextual. What is clear, however, is that humans are increasingly identified as responsible for environmental change. Our ongoing "alterations to climate, water, land and ecosystems. . . [are] challenging all life on our planet, with serious implications for human health" (Lancet Planetary Health 2017, p. e1). This human responsibility, and the inevitability that humans will experience the impacts of inaction, is the essence of the contemporary concept of planetary health.

A Focus on Climate Change and Its Impact on Health in Australia

Although arguably just one process impacting the health of the planet and the health of those who inhabit it, the principal focus for this chapter is climate change. This is justified firstly by the sheer impact of climate instability both now and into the future. Secondly, climate change presents a test case for the reaction of the human race to a life-threatening problem for our planet. Thirdly, Australia is "highly vulnerable to climate change", by virtue of its unique and fragile geoclimatic environment (Hanna and McIver 2018, p. 312).

'Climate change' is a broad term used to describe a series of changes to the earth's climate system that persist for several decades or longer. The properties of the climate that change include averages, variability and extremes. Historically, these changes have been the result of natural processes, such as changes in the sun's radiation. More recently, the evidence is clear that climate change is the result of human-induced activities, particularly the burning of fossil fuels and mass deforestation. These practices have led to increases in the amount of greenhouse gases in the earth's atmosphere (particularly carbon dioxide), which in turn impacts on the temperature regulation that keeps our planet habitable.

There are numerous biophysical effects from this process. Further, they are complicated because the fragile nature of the earth's climate system ensures they are all, in some way, interrelated. A disturbance to one aspect of the climate system can trigger changes in other systems, which can be either immediate or take years to become apparent. The changes expected to adversely impact Australia can be classified into five basic processes:

- Increased temperature averages and variability
- Increased regularity of extreme weather events leading to natural hazards, such as heatwave, drought, flood, tsunami and cyclone events
- Increased disease from vector populations, such as mosquitoes
- Rising sea levels leading to displacement in coastal zones

Reporting on the 'Angry Summer' of 2016/2017, the Climate Council of Australia lists record-breaking temperatures in the nation's major cities, powerful bushfire events and unprecedented storm and flooding activity (Steffen et al. 2017). The impacts of climate change on the health of many Australians are therefore already very real. The following section is a rapid review of some of the primary pathways for harm associated with our changing climate. Given that heat "represents Australia's greatest current climate-related health burden" (Hanna and McIver 2018, p. 312), we start there.

Rising Temperatures and Heatwaves

The human body has limits to the extent it can adapt to excessively high temperatures, and Australians should be prepared to endure more regular extreme heat events in the future. More alarmingly, these events are pre-dicted to be increasingly prolonged and intense. Potential health impacts of heatwaves include minor rashes and body cramps, dehydration and sleep disturbances. At its most extreme, heat can lead to conditions requiring hospitalisation, such as heatstroke, which can result in death. The frail elderly, the very young, those with disabilities, those suffering from chronic disease and those in low socio-economic groups are most at risk. The impact of increased temperatures is exacerbated in Australia's cities by the urban heat island effect. This is a phenomenon of microcli-mate change where, primarily as a result of the sheer concentration of heat-retaining built form, cities are several degrees hotter than surround-ing non-urbanised land. Urban heat islands struggle to follow the pro-cess of nocturnal cooling that characterises natural ecosystems. This is an emergent, yet deeply concerning, outcome of climate change in Australia because it impacts 67% of us who live in major cities (Australian Bureau of Statistics 2017). The increased incidence of extreme heat events is an example of the way the causes and health impacts of climate change are interrelated and reinforcing. Higher temperatures increase demand for cool spaces, which are usually achieved using energy-intensive air-conditioning units. The carbon emitted in this process further contributes to climate change, which in turn raises the temperature.

Drought

Extended periods of below-average rainfall are known as droughts. The immediate health impacts of these events are related to reduced water supply and decreased air quality, which can affect respiratory health and hygiene. Immediate effects are also felt by farming communities where drought means an abrupt drop in revenue, thereby limiting discretionary income available for all but the necessities. Droughts also increase the risk of bushfire which threatens human health in various ways discussed below. It is, however, the long-term impacts of drought that have the most damaging health impacts. Australian surveys prove that farmers experiencing drought are more likely to report mental health problems, and that drought is associated with an increased relative risk of suicide, particularly among men aged 30–49 (Australian Institute of Health and Welfare 2018).

Bushfires

Although the Australian bush relies on periods of intense burning for processes of regeneration, the frequency and intensity of bushfires in Aus-tralia are increasing, as is the impact on the health of the population. Between 1967 and 2013, bushfires in Australia accounted for 433 deaths and more than 8,000 injuries (Geoscience Australia 2018). Other health impacts associated with bushfires include increased incidence of respiratory and heart problems, such as asthma and chronic obstructive pulmonary disease, as well as psychological trauma, destruction of property, livestock and wildlife, and long-term contamination of water sources.

Air Pollution

Many of the health impacts associated with poor air quality are not directly the result of climate change. However, increased temperatures and extreme weather events do expose the population to episodes of severe air pollution. The smoke and haze associated with bushfires are the most obvious examples. However, there are also respiratory illness impacts from changes in air quality associated with thunderstorms. The term 'thunderstorm asthma' has been used to describe asthma triggered by an uncommon combination of high pollen and a particular type of thunderstorm. An event in the State of Victoria in 2016 resulted in a 58% increase in presentations to public hospital emergency departments and nine deaths (Australian Institute of Health and Welfare 2018). The incidence of thunderstorm asthma events reported in Australia is increasing.

Sea Level Rise

Sea level rise is a consequence of both thermal expansion related to increased sea temperatures and melting ice sheets and glaciers. This is of concern to Australia given that much of our urban development is along the coastal fringe (Gurran et al. 2011). Damage to homes and critical infrastructure is one of the predicted outcomes, with health impacts ranging from injury from eroded and unstable coastlines to loss of community fabric and financial hardship. Sea level rise also has enormous implications for our neighbours in the low-lying islands of the South Pacific, threatening to displace thousands.

This chapter has so far provided a brief introduction to the complex concept of planetary health and used climate change to demonstrate some of the key pathways between depletion of the biophysical environment and human health. The case is simple and compelling—planetary ill health must be considered a key risk factor for human health. There are direct and indirect health consequences of climate change, all of which impact on risk factors for chronic disease and our response to creating health-supportive built environments. Social, cultural and economic factors, particularly access to financial resources, will further complicate and exacerbate the health implications of climate change (see Figure 3.1). We now turn to exploring some of the ways urban planning in Australia can be used to protect and promote the health of the planet, again using climate change as our point of reference.

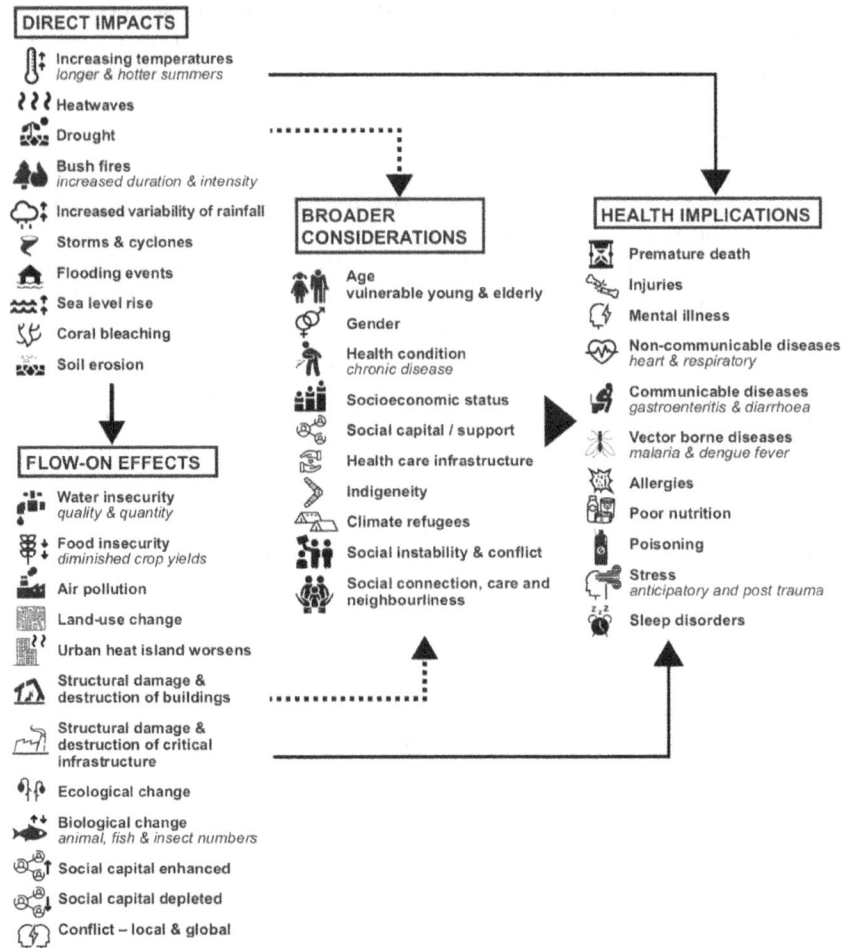

Figure 3.1 The impacts of climate change on health

Source: Adapted from: Horsburgh et al. 2017; Watts et al. 2015

Planning for Planetary Health Protection from an Australian Perspective

The vastness of the Australian continent and its accompanying ecological diversity pose particular challenges for coordinated responses to climate change and the health of the planet more generally. In many ways, it is deeply concerning for us to acknowledge that, to date, Australia's response to climate change has been fragmented, piecemeal and, at best, tokenistic. Notably absent has been a lack of respect for different types of knowledge, especially that of the community and Aboriginal and Torres Strait Islander people. Rhetoric on the need for integrative solutions and interdisciplinary approaches to climate change in Australia abounds. Any realisation of this is largely illusory, with power invested in professional specialisations, conflicts of interest between different government portfolios, a market-led (neo-liberal) planning system and disparate political goals.

The International Setting

Internationally, a range of key initiatives have set the context for Australia's policy and practice in relation to the health of the planet. Concerns about environmental degradation across the globe have been growing since the middle of the 20th Century. The World Commission on Environment and Development, in its report *Our Common Future*, first used the term 'sustainable development' in 1987, proposing a new 'human/environment relationship' to balance 'environmental integrity and human well-being' (World Commission on Environment and Development 1987 in Brown 2001). A few years later, in 1992, Agenda 21 emerged from the United Nation's Earth Summit Conference in Rio de Janeiro, Brazil, linking environmental sustainability and human health (Barton and Tsourou 2000). The undertakings made during this seminal meeting were revisited 20 years later at Rio+20. Political, professional and community representatives from across the globe reaffirmed their commitment to sustainable development for the planet's future and the world's population (United Nations [UN] 2012). This was formalised in the policy document 'The Future We Want', which sets out the foundations of the global Sustainability Development Goals. These goals are enshrined in the 2030 Agenda for Sustainable Development, which lists Good Health and Wellbeing as its third goal (UN 2015).

Concerns about climate change as a specific issue have now occupied the international scene for some time. The Intergovernmental Panel on Climate Change was established in 1988 under the auspices of the United Nations Environment Programme and the World Meteorological Organization. There have now been five assessment reports, with the first published in 1990 and the most recent in 2014 (Intergovernmental Panel on Climate Change 2015). The Intergovernmental Panel has been controversial, and although based on scientific evidence, many governments have derided the dire predictions and calls for action. Finally, in 2015, we had progress, with the signing of the Paris Agreement under the United Nations Framework Convention on Climate Change. This is the UN entity that manages and, under the 2015 Agreement, monitors the global response to climate change (United Nations Climate Change 2018).

The Australian Government Response

So how is Australia addressing climate change in the context of protecting the planet's health? It is inevitably a multilayered response, reflecting the country's governance arrangements (see Chapter 1—Australia and Australia's Planning). But before we consider these complexities, it is important to note that prior to white settlement, our Aboriginal and Torres Strait Islander people lived in harmony with Australia's fragile biophysical environment. Until recently, much of this intimate climatic knowledge and adaptive capacity had been ignored, to the detriment of Australia's biodiversity, atmosphere and its fragile ecosystems (McKenzie 2017). Encouragingly, this deep ecological wisdom is slowly being recognised, in part for the way in which it focuses attention on the intrinsic value of the environment (Baum 2008).

National

Action to address climate change in Australia has emerged from the broader framework of environmental sustainability. Mandated under the Commonwealth's *Environment Protection and Biodiversity Conservation Act* 1999, State of Environment reporting is a method for assessing national progress on environmental management and identifying emerging issues needing attention. At the national level, this is conducted every five years via an independent, expert-driven and evidence-based review (Jackson et al. 2017).

Since 2011, climate change has been routinely examined as part of State of Environment reporting. In the context of the impact of heat, the need for a comprehensive national approach to reducing greenhouse gas emissions has been affirmed, together with climate change mitigation and adaptation more broadly. In the context of urban air quality, concerns for human health have also been identified (Department of the Environment and Energy 2018b). In the latest report (2016), it was noted that climate change posed significant risks for health as a result of increasing temperatures and related events, such as higher levels of air pollution and heatwaves.

In 2018, the Australian government's response to climate change occurs through the Federal Department of the Environment and Energy (Department of the Environment and Energy 2018a). In relation to climate change, Australia is a signatory to the Paris Agreement. The Federal government ratified the agreement in November 2016, establishing a target of reducing GHG emissions by 26–28% below the nation's 2005 emission levels by 2030 (Department of Foreign Affairs and Trade 2015).

State

We outlined in Chapter 1 that our nation is comprised of six States and two Territories, which regulate different aspects of the governance of Australia. Mirroring the State of the Environment reporting by the

Table 3.2 Climate change policies at the State level in Australia

State	Policy
ACT	*AP2: A new climate change strategy and action plan for the Australian Capital Territory*: www.environment.act.gov.au/cc
New South Wales	*NSW Climate Change Policy Framework*: www.environment.nsw.gov.au/topics/climate-change/policy-framework
Northern Territory	None at present
Queensland	*Pathways to a clean growth economy: Queensland Climate Transition Strategy*: www.qld.gov.au/environment/climate/transition
South Australia	*Change Strategy 2015–2050—Towards a low carbon economy*: www.environment.sa.gov.au/Science/Science_research/climate-change/climate-change-initiatives-in-south-australia/sa-climate-change-strategy
Tasmania	*Climate Action 21: Tasmania's Climate Change Action Plan 2017–2021*: www.dpac.tas.gov.au/divisions/climatechange/tasmanias_climate_change_action_plan_20172021
Victoria	*Climate Change Framework*: www.climatechange.vic.gov.au/victorias-climate-change-framework
Western Australia	*Adapting to our changing climate*: www.der.wa.gov.au/your-environment/climate-change/255-publications-and-resources

URLs accessed 17 May 2018

Commonwealth government, the States and Territories also undertake similar methodical and detailed monitoring of the environment. The particular policies that focus on climate change, including the health effects of climate change, are listed in Table 3.2.

Local

Local government is the nation's third tier of government and is most in touch with the needs of local communities. Indeed, this is the scale of government where a majority of the safeguards to protect the population against the health impacts of climate change are enacted. Local governments in Australia are responsible for planning for bushfire protection, attempting to mitigate the urban heat island effect by greening our urban areas (see Figure 3.2) and accommodating the coastal erosion predicted to accompany sea level rise (see Box 3.1). Local authorities are also involved in the management of hazard reduction burns and the provision of assistance to families and individuals experiencing natural disasters.

Given the extreme regional variability of climate change impacts across the vast Australian continent, the importance of an in-depth appreciation of local demographic, sociocultural, environmental and built form characteristics cannot be overstated in any attempt to protect the health of the community. Although increasingly constrained by State directives, Local government retains a significant role in urban planning, both in the preparation of strategic plans for future land use and the approval of building plans for new developments. It is critical that prospects for climate change mitigation and adaptation are embedded in both of these endeavours.

Box 3.1   Protecting Australia's coastal regions from the impacts of climate change

The urgent need for targeted and coordinated actions to address the implications of climate change–associated coastal erosion and sea level rise is recognised across Australia. Queensland's QCoast2100 is an example of a program designed to assist coastal councils in Queensland do just this. By providing funding, tools and technical support, QCoast2100 aims to assist in key areas of operation, such as:

- Land use planning and development assessment
- Infrastructure planning and management, including roads, storm water and foreshore protection
- Asset management and planning, including nature conservation, recreation, cultural heritage values and other public amenities
- Community planning
- Emergency management

As well as enabling an immediate response, the program addresses longer-term professional capacity building and the development of networks across all sectors so that Local government can effectively engage with the private sector, researchers and higher levels of government in responding to climate change impacts along the coastal region (QCoast2100 2018).

Aimed at a broader national audience, CoastAdapt is an Australia-wide resource (Coast Adapt 2018). It brings together a vast compendium of information and guidance to manage the multiple and complex range of risks posed by climate change along the coastline. The web-based resource contains basic information and educational tools, and a comprehensive decision support framework for assessing coastal climate change–related risks. Detailed health impacts are presented on one of the site's 'Impact Sheets' (Bambrick 2016).

How have health and built environment professionals responded?

The Health Profession

Tony McMichael, the eminent Australian epidemiologist, was responsible for internationally seminal work identifying the direct and indirect impacts of global warming on population health (see Butler et al. 2015 for a comprehensive overview of McMichael's work). McMichael differentiated the catastrophic implications—such as more frequent bushfires and cyclones—of climate change events from the ongoing and wider consequences of rising temperatures and changing rainfall patterns. He stated that both physical and mental health will be adversely affected, both directly in terms of acute diseases and indirectly in terms of the exacerbation of chronic conditions. McMichael's contribution was instrumental in recognising the complex nature of health impacts due to climate change (see Figure 3.1). He researched how this would affect crop production, economic productivity, social stability, peaceful global cooperation, poor communities, and vulnerable groups such as the young, disabled and elderly.

McMichael's work has long been championed by Tony Capon, another leading Australian public health professional, who has worked in both practitioner and researcher roles. In 2017, Capon was appointed the inaugural Professor of Planetary Health at The University of Sydney. This is a world first and confirms that the concept of planetary health is becoming an accepted way of conceptualising the human role in the protection of the earth's fragile ecosystem. Capon's focus is on the health implications of urbanisation from an interdisciplinary perspective, employing systems approaches to understand the complex web of interactions and relationships between the built environment and health.

Operating at the policy level, healthcare professionals from the fields of medicine, nursing, public health, social work and psychology, alongside healthcare service providers, researchers and consumers, come together in a voluntary coalition called the Climate and Health Alliance, whose mission is the development of policy to address climate change–related health threats to both humans and the environment (Climate and Health Alliance 2018). In 2017, the coalition released an overarching framework, urging the development of a comprehensive national policy to address health risks of climate change, focusing on equity and environmental sustainability (see Table 3.2).

The Australian Medical Association (AMA) and the Royal Australian College of Physicians (RACP) have also both issued comprehensive position statements informing their members of the issues and urging ongoing education about the implications of climate change for health (Australian Medical Association 2004; Royal Australian College of Physicians 2018). It is also encouraging to see that in 2018, the AMA devoted a

Table 3.3 National climate change policy framework and principles

National climate change policy framework action areas:	National climate change policy framework principles:
• Health-promoting and emissions-reducing policies • Emergency and disaster preparedness • Support for healthy and resilient communities • Education and capacity building • Leadership and governance • Sustainable and climate-resilient health sector • Research and data	• The right to health • Community safety and resilience • Environmental protection as a foundation for health and wellbeing • Health in All Policies • Intragenerational and intergenerational equity • Minimising and managing risk • Indigenous rights, recognition and reconciliation • Citizen engagement

Source: Horsburgh et al. 2017

special issue of its members' *Medical Journal of Australia* to the topic of planetary health. Nevertheless, there is little discussion about the need to work with other professions, especially those in the built environment, to address the situation.

Finally, it is pertinent to note that the Australian Institute of Health and Welfare's comprehensive biennial report on the nation's health status has, for the first time, included a full chapter on the relationship between the environment and human health (Australian Institute of Health and Welfare 2018). Entitled 'Impacts of the natural environment on health', this chapter discusses how our physical and mental health is affected by a broad range of environmental factors, with a particular focus on climate change. There is coverage of a range of government policies and community programs aimed at preventing and managing the identified environmental health consequences. The inclusion of environment and health in this national and authoritative compendium is a further acknowledgement of the importance of the planetary–human health nexus.

The Planning Profession

Although we maintain that the terminology around the planning–planetary health relationship is a recent one, Australia's urban planners have a long-standing interest in the protection of the planet, including the need to address climate change and its impacts. This interest has waxed and waned along with the need for planners to balance competing agendas and work within the constraints of the planning system. Perhaps as a wake-up call to the profession, in 2001, Valerie Brown—one of the nation's most eminent sustainability and systems researchers—used the Australian Planning Institute's national peer-reviewed journal to ask planning practitioners whether they still had a role in "reforming the people/planet relationship" (Brown 2001, p. 67). Here, she spoke of the pending collapse of global life support systems before the middle of the 21st Century and the fragmented ways of working in Australia to address these issues. This gloomy outlook was tempered by her assertions of the potential for planners to "contribute to a sustainable and humane future through their capacities to consult, to predict, to be strategic and to provide holistic direction" (Brown 2001, p. 67).

In general, Australian built environment researchers, policymakers and practitioners have made significant contributions to enhancing the health of the planet in their varied responses to climate change. Research-led organisations have brought academics together in a range of cooperative and multidisciplinary bodies. The National Climate Change Adaptation Research Facility, based in Queensland at Griffith University, is one such example. First established in 2008, this facility's mission is to provide research evidence for policy and decision-makers managing climate change risk. Its recent focus has been on Australia's expansive coastal zone, principally to assist Local governments in responding to climate change impacts, including flooding and coastal erosion. Supported by the Australian Federal government, the Cooperative Research Centre for Low Carbon Living is another research entity with a broad remit to consider social, technological and policy levers to reduce greenhouse gas emissions in the built environment. The development of low carbon building construction materials and associated tools and technologies, progressing the evidence base for government policy, planning and practice initiatives and engaging communities in low carbon living are key goals (Low Carbon Living CRC 2018).

Commitment to protecting the planet from the impacts of climate change is evident across built environment practitioners, including overarching peak bodies in the sector. The Australian Sustainable Built Environment Council brings together different organisations involved in the planning, design and construction of the built environment to advocate for sustainability via different policies and practices (Australian Sustainable Built Environment Council 2018). The Green Building Council of Australia is another active organisation in this space, maintaining four Green Star rating tools available for certification of design, construction and operation of buildings, fitouts and communities. The program is voluntary and covers residential, office, retail, accommodation, education and public buildings (Green Building Council Australia 2018). Specific professional associations also have established commitments to addressing climate change. In 2015, the Planning Institute of Australia (PIA) issued a position statement affirming the national planning body's acceptance of the science that human activity is responsible for altering the world's climate, that there is already irreversible change, and that planning professionals have a responsibility to work to address this reality (Planning Institute of Australia 2015). As well as acknowledging the uneven impact of climate change on the Australian continent and different communities, PIA voices its concern about the absence of "long-term strategic leadership", which underpins Australia's "fragmented policy response".

Community Response

There has been a long history of involvement of the Australian people with their environment. For example, early chapters in this book have explored Indigenous stewardship of the land, and how this has been largely eschewed since the very recent arrival of white Europeans just over 200 years ago. We cannot begin to do justice to such an historical legacy here, but we do want to mention how contemporary communities are engaging with environmental protection, particularly in relation to addressing climate change.

As community members vote for governments and comprise the professional ranks, they have had a say in the responses discussed above. However, there are myriad specific community-based groups advocating in different ways for a strong response to combat climate change to protect both the planet's health and that of the population. Groups can be focused on a local activity, such as community gardening or fighting a specific proposal for a development deemed to have the potential to cause dire environmental consequences. In terms of climate change response, there are some national entities who host web platforms to inform the community at large. HOPE Australia (Householders' Options to Protect the Environment) is one such organisation. It has a resource-rich website (HOPE Australia 2012) that includes contacts for non-government organisations, government and businesses involved in planetary protection. Act on Climate Now (2018) is an organisation established to assist independent climate action community groups on the ground across Australia. Solar Citizens is an independent community group that advocates for the use and support of solar energy across Australia given its plentiful sunshine (Solar Citizens 2018). More broadly, organisations such as OzGreen (OzGreen 2018) focus on education to enable people to take action to protect the environment. This group has a strong focus on young people's involvement, skill development and networks.

A more formal community organisation, the Climate Council, is an independent, crowd-funded organisation that reports on the nation's climate change response. It is very telling that the council asserts that Australia's performance in tackling climate change is seriously wanting on every level: "Amongst the G20 countries, Australia's emissions-reduction target—a reduction of 26–28% on a 2005 baseline—is unusually weak, nowhere near what is required for us to play our fair share in tackling climate change" (Steffen et al. 2017). Political will and courageous leadership, together with vested interests, have played a role in undermining the establishment of a coherent national climate change policy (Steffen et al. 2017).

An Integrative Approach—The Co-Benefits

Climate change has the potential to destabilise the planet's health in a way that will be catastrophic. This, in turn, will have devastating impacts on human health across the globe. Almost 20 years into the 21st Century, there are fewer denials about the threats that a changing climate can pose, but concerted, committed and integrated action across the political spectrum remains elusive. In this chapter, which focuses on the disciplines of health and the built environment, we have shown how Australian governments and professionals are proceeding. Nevertheless, there is more to be done, especially in integrating our response to ensure the planet's future health. In this final section, we look at how this can be achieved using the co-benefits framework. This is an approach in which a particular action addressing climate change brings about multiple and unanticipated benefits across different sectors, including the community.

A good example of the co-benefits approach in action is active transport, conceptualised in this book as walking and cycling. We cover the benefits and barriers associated with active transport in Chapter Four—Planning for Physical Activity. In short, active transport enables mobility that is both healthy for the individual and better for the environment. For example, when people walk or cycle rather than drive, carbon dioxide emissions are reduced, which in turn is positive for respiratory and heart health, as is being physically active. Vehicular traffic congestion is reduced, and local businesses benefit, as there are more people out and about, connecting with each other in safe and socially vibrant communities. This demonstrates the way a policy to enhance the provision of active transport options has multiple benefits that flow to the environment, economy, human health and society in general. The provision of green infrastructure is another case in point, and this relationship is demonstrated in Figure 3.2.

Australian researchers are investigating different ways to advance the use of co-benefits. With funding through the Cooperative Research Centre for Low Carbon Living, Melbourne University's Mark Stevenson, an epidemiologist who bridges urban transport and public health, is leading a project to develop a co-benefits calculator. This will be used to assist decision-making by stakeholders in the public and private sectors, as well as community members, enabling the measurement of health and productivity outcomes of a policy proposal. It is anticipated that the calculator will be linked to built environment features, such as residential characteristics, mixed uses, open space and active transport provisions, and the configuration of the local street network. Hilary Bambrick, who heads up the Queensland University of Technology's

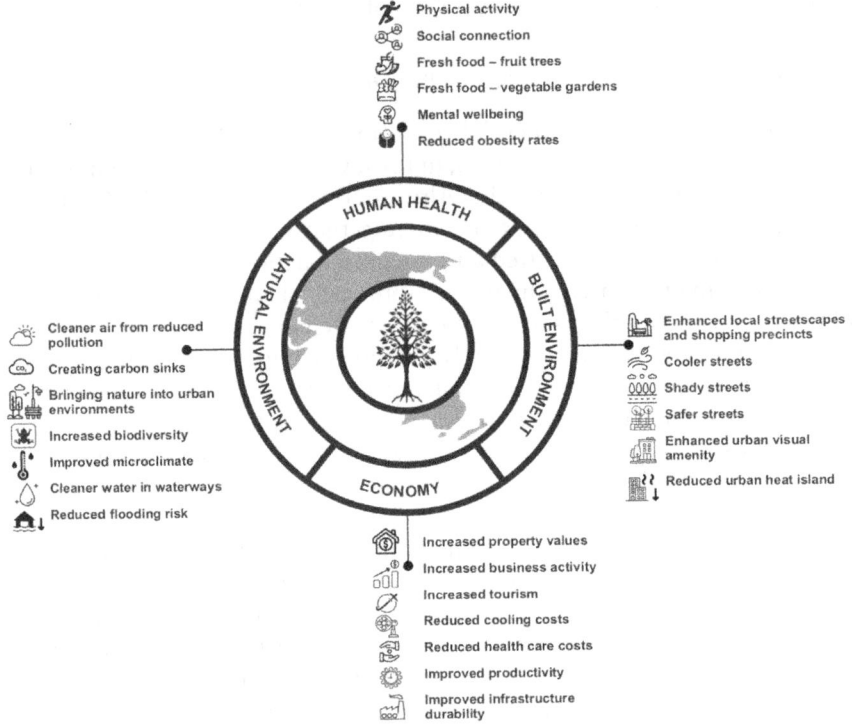

Figure 3.2 The co-benefits of green infrastructure

Source: Adapted from AECOM 2017; Government Architect NSW 2017

School of Public Health and Social Work, has also contributed to our understanding of how to look through a 'co-benefits lens' in addressing the health implications of climate change (Bambrick et al. 2011). In particular, she has shown how a connected and strong community can be more resilient to the impacts of climate change. For example, the ability to produce food in local communities is a practice of resilience and reduces the carbon emissions associated with the transport of food. Concurrently, this practice can increase physical activity and access to fresh food as well as develop social cohesion as neighbours are brought together in the process. This, in turn, can enhance community resilience in the event of a catastrophic climate event such as a prolonged heatwave, flood or bushfire.

A final and striking example of the co-benefits of addressing climate change and health is the dire need to address the climate change–fuelled hot urban environment, with its associated negative consequences for human and planetary health. Penrith City Council, in the oft-scorching western region of the Sydney metropolis, has developed a cooling strategy, which showcases how this can be achieved (see Box 3.2).

Box 3.2   Penrith's Cooling the City Strategy

On 7 January 2018, the suburban area of Penrith, located in Sydney's outer west, recorded the hottest temperature (47.3 degrees Celsius) of any place on earth on that day (McInnes 2018). While this was an extreme event, in terms of metropolitan Sydney, the microclimate of the Penrith region is hotter and drier.

For some time now, Penrith City Council has been concerned about the impact of urban heat, rising temperatures and more frequent, extreme weather events. This motivated the Council's adoption of a cooling strategy in 2015 (Penrith City Council 2015). The strategy identifies particular climatic challenges for the 200,000 residents of Penrith, who face more hot days over summer and less cool nights. The topography of the area means that it does not benefit from sea breezes, which bring summer temperatures down along Sydney's eastern seaboard.

Using the overarching themes of community engagement, collaboration, sustainability and efficiency, the cooling strategy sets out specific actions to help the community adapt to increased heat in the 21st Century. Based on the evidence that heat poses significant financial, environmental and social risks, the threat to health is especially concerning. The strategy identifies vulnerable groups, who face specific difficulties adjusting to heat because of economic disadvantage, social situation, health status or age. Heat will also have an adverse impact on liveability. The strategy notes that vegetation—both grass and trees—and water bodies are important in mitigating heat and have significant co-benefits.

The cooling strategy identifies three main actions for managing urban heat, broadly identifying them as 'green' and 'non-green':

1. Green infrastructure
2. Water sensitive urban design (WSUD)
3. Increased albedo/reflectivity

Green infrastructure includes both designed and natural vegetation, such as parks, recreation areas, remnant vegetation, residential gardens, street trees, community gardens and so-called "greening technologies" like green rooftops and building walls. These are the types of green infrastructure from which a raft of co-benefits flow:

- Flood alleviation and management
- Storm water quality improvement
- Improved physical and mental health
- Habitat and biodiversity benefits
- Enhancement of public spaces
- Opportunities for recreation and leisure
- Support of economic growth, productivity, investment and local tourism
- Opportunities for urban agriculture

Important co-benefits are also evident through increasing albedo (or reflectivity) of materials to reduce their absorption of heat, demanding a shift to lighter-coloured materials for paving and roofing. These co-benefits are identified in the strategy and include better night-time visibility and longevity of roads and footpaths. In turn, this improves the economic situation of the council, enabling spending in other areas.

Penrith's Cooling the City Strategy informs other policies, such as environmental sustainability, and controls for development and design. In addition, it engages the community through education about heat risks and mitigation approaches.

Source: Penrith City Council 2015

While Australia's urban planners have accepted their role in reducing climate change impacts, there is still a way to go in getting urban planners to embrace health promotion as a primary outcome of their work. Adopting a co-benefits approach provides a positive way forward. It demonstrates the way a well-accepted policy action in one disciplinary domain can have multiple and broader benefits.

Conclusion

A healthy planet is the basis for all life. Without a healthy planet, there is no life, let alone the possibility of a healthy built environment supporting people's health and wellness. Protecting the planet's health is complex, particularly in the 21st Century, as we witness both the way our climate is changing and the potentially dire consequences. Dealing with the direct impacts on our health, the associated flow-on effects and the uneven distribution of these further exacerbates this complexity.

In this chapter, we have presented the case for considering the destruction of the planet a risk factor for human health. We have provided a broad overview of Australia's response to protecting its environment, focusing our attention on the most pressing of contemporary challenges—that of climate change. This discussion has revealed a mixed set of actions amidst growing concern about the direct and indirect impacts on the health of Australians, particularly those with the least ability to adjust and adapt. As a prosperous and developed nation, Australia has a responsibility to the global community, as well as its own peoples, to address the impact of climate change as well as other environmental problems. The need to work across the disciplines of health and the built environment has been highlighted, along with the potential of the co-benefits approach to achieve other goals in a range of jurisdictions.

References

Act on Climate Now (2018) *Act on Climate Now: A Democratic Non-Profit Community Organisation*, www.aoc.org.au/ [Accessed 29 July 2018].

AECOM (2017) *Green Infrastructure: A Vital Step to Brilliant Australian Cities*, AECOM, Sydney, NSW.

Australian Bureau of Statistics (2017) *Australian Demographic Statistics, June 2017*, Cat. no. 3101.0, Australian Bureau of Statistics, Canberra.

Australian Institute of Health and Welfare (2018) *Australia's Health 2018*, Australian Institute of Health and Welfare, Canberra.

Australian Medical Association (2004) *Climate Change and Human Health*, revised 2008 and 2015, https://ama.com.au/position-statement/ama-position-statement-climate-change-and-human-health-2004-revised-2015 [Accessed 29 July 2018].

Australian Sustainable Built Environment Council (2018) *About Us*, www.asbec.asn.au/about-us/ [Accessed 29 July 2018].

Bambrick, H. J. (2016) *Climate Change Impacts on Human Health in the Coastal Zone*, Impact Sheet 5, National Climate Change Adaptation Research Facility, Gold Coast.

Bambrick, H. J., Capon, A. G., Barnett, G. B., Beaty, R. M. and Burton, A. J. (2011) Climate change and health in the Urban environment: Adaptation opportunities in Australian cities. *Asia-Pacific Journal of Public Health*, 23(2) Suppl. pp. 67S–79S.

Barton, H. and Grant, M. (2006) A health map for the local human habitat. *Journal of the Royal Society for the Promotion of Health*, 126(6) pp. 252–253.

Barton, H. and Tsourou, C. (2000) *Healthy Urban Planning: A WHO Guide to Planning for People*, Spon, London.

Baum, F. (2008) *The New Public Health*, 3rd edition, Oxford University Press, Oxford.

Brown, V. (2001) Planners and the Planet: Reforming the people/planet relationship: Do planners have a role? *Australian Planner*, 38(2) pp. 67–73.

Butler, C., Dixon, J. and Capon, T. eds. (2015) *Health of People, Places and Planet. Reflections Based on Tony McMichael's Four Decades of Contribution to Epidemiological Understanding*, ANU Press, Acton, ACT.

Climate and Health Alliance (2018) *About*, www.caha.org.au/about [Accessed 29 July 2018].

Coast Adapt (2018) *A Changing Climate in Coastal Australia: Build Knowledge, Take Action*, https://coastadapt.com.au/ [Accessed 29 July 2018].

Department of the Environment and Energy (2018a) *About Us*, Department of the Environment and Energy, Australian Government, www.environment.gov.au/about-us [Accessed 29 July 2018].

Department of the Environment and Energy (2018b) *State of the Environment (SoE) Reporting Themes: Atmosphere*, Department of the Environment and Energy, Australian Government, http://155.187.2.69/soe/themes/atmosphere.html [Accessed 29 July 2018].

Department of Foreign Affairs and Trade (2015) *Australia's Intended Nationally Determined Contribution to a New Climate Change Agreement*, August, Department of Foreign Affairs and Trade, Australian Government, Canberra.

Geoscience Australia (2018) *Bushfire*, Geoscience Australia, Australian Government, Canberra, www.ga.gov.au/scientific-topics/hazards/bushfire [Accessed 29 July 2018].

Government Architect NSW (2017) *Greener Places*, Draft Policy, NSW Government, Sydney, NSW.

Green Building Council Australia (2018) *Rating System*, https://new.gbca.org.au/green-star/rating-system/ [Accessed 29 July 2018].

Gurran, N., Norman, B., Gilbert, C. and Hamin, E. (2011) *Planning for Climate Change Adaptation in Coastal Australia: State of Practice*, Report No. 4 for the National Sea Change Taskforce, University of Sydney.

Hanna, E. G. and McIver, L. J. (2018) Climate change: A brief overview of the science and health impacts for Australia. *Medical Journal of Australia*, 208(7) pp. 311–315.

HOPE Australia (2012) *HOPE Australia: Householder's Options to Protect the Environment (HOPE) Inc*, www.hopeaustralia.org.au/ [Accessed 29 July 2018].

Horsburgh, N., Armstrong, F. and Mulvenna, V. (2017) *Framework for a National Strategy on Climate Change, Health and Well-Being for Australia*, Climate and Health Alliance, Melbourne.

Intergovernmental Panel on Climate Change (2015) *IPCC Factsheet: Timeline–Highlights of IPCC History*, IPCC Secretariat, Geneva, www.ipcc.ch/news_and_events/docs/factsheets/FS_timeline.pdf [Accessed 29 July 2018].

Jackson, W. J., Argent, R. M., Bax, N. J., Clark, G. F., Coleman, S., Cresswell, I. D., Emmerson, K. M., Evans, K., Hibberd, M. F., Johnston, E. L., et al. (2017) *Australia: State of the Environment, 2016*, Department of the Environment and Energy, Australian Government, Canberra.

The Lancet Planetary Health (2017) Welcome to *The Lancet Planetary Health*. *The Lancet Planetary Health*, 1(1) p. e1.

Low Carbon Living CRC (2018) *National Research and Innovation Hub for the Built Environment*, www.lowcarbonlivingcrc.com.au/ [Accessed 29 July 2018].

McInnes, W. (2018) Sydney clocks the hottest place on Earth as hot weather continues. *Sydney Morning Herald*, 8 January 2018, www.smh.com.au [Accessed 29 July 2018].

McKenzie, L. (2017) *Design, Context and Use of Public Space: The Influence of Heat on Everyday Behaviour in Outdoor Settings–A Western Sydney Case*

Study, Unpublished PhD Thesis, Faculty of Built Environment, UNSW, Sydney, NSW.

OzGREEN (2018) *What We Do*, www.ozgreen.org/what_we_do [Accessed 29 July 2018].

Penrith City Council (2015) *Cooling the City Strategy*, August, Penrith City Council, Penrith, NSW.

Planning Institute of Australia (2015) *Planning in a Changing Climate Position Statement August 2015*, www.planning.org.au/policy/climate-change-0815/planning-in-a-changing-climate-position-statement-august-2015 [Accessed 29 July 2018].

QCoast2100 (2018) *About QCoast2100*, www.qcoast2100.com.au/about [Accessed 29 July 2018].

Rockström, J., Steffen, W., Noone, K., Persson, Å., Chapin, F. S., Lambin, E. F., Lenton, T. M., Scheffer, M., Folke, C., Schellnhuber, H. J., et al. (2009) A safe operating space for humanity. *Nature*, 461 pp. 472–475.

Royal Australian College of Physicians (2018) *Climate Change and Health*, www.racp.edu.au/fellows/resources/curated-collections/climate-change-and-health [Accessed 29 July 2018].

Solar Citizen (2018) *Solar Citizens*, www.solarcitizens.org.au/ [Accessed 29 July 2018].

Steffen, W., Richardon, K., Rockström, J., Cornell, S., Fetzer, I., Bennet, E. M., Biggs, R., Carpenter, S. R., de Vries, W., de Wit, C. A., et al. (2015) Planetary boundaries: Guiding human development on a changing planet. *Science*, 347(6223) pp. 1259855-1–1259855-10.

Steffen, W., Stock, A., Alexander, D. and Rice, M. (2017) *Angry Summer 2016/17: Climate Change Super-Charging Extreme Weather*, Climate Council, Potts Point, NSW.

Thompson, S. M. and Capon, A. (2015) The co-benefits framework for understanding and action on climate change, in Barton, H., Thompson, S., Grant, M. and Burgess, S. eds., *The Routledge Handbook of Planning for Health and Well-Being: Shaping a Sustainable and Healthy Future*, Routledge, London, pp. 319–332.

United Nations (2012) *The Future We Want*, resolution A/66/288, United Nations, New York.

United Nations (2015) *Transforming Our World: The 2030 Agenda for Sustainable Development*, resolution A/RES/70/1, United Nations, New York.

United Nations Climate Change (2018) *About the Secretariat*, https://unfccc.int/about-us/about-the-secretariat [Accessed 29 July 2018].

Watts, N., Adger, W. N., Agnolucci, P., Blackstock, J., Byass, P., Cai, W., Chaytor, S., Colbourn, T., Collins, M., Cooper, A., et al. (2015) Health and climate change: Policy responses to protect public health. *Lancet*, 386 pp. 1861–1914.

4 Planning for Physical Activity

Introduction

Physical activity is any bodily movement that exerts the muscles of the body. All bodily movement is therefore a form of physical activity, whether it is washing the car, walking to the shops or train station, going to the gym or playing a sport.

Australia's built environments support physical activity in different ways. These include designing street networks and providing infrastructure for walking and cycling for both recreation and transport. Decreasing the distances we need to travel by mixing uses and increasing densities also promotes physical activity by encouraging walking and cycling for transport. The provision and preservation of plentiful open spaces for recreational use are other critically important factors. This chapter addresses all of these issues in the Australian context, starting with a review of the importance of physical activity.

Why is Physical Activity Important?

Being active enables participation in daily life and is a key component of human flourishing. Physical activity helps us maintain a healthy weight and lowers vulnerability to many of the most common and costly chronic diseases facing Australia, including coronary heart disease, diabetes and cancer. Children and young people need physical activity to develop both physically and cognitively. Being active is proven to lower the risk of many mental illnesses, including depression, and declines in cognitive function as we age. Furthermore, physical activity, particularly weight-bearing activity, is a key factor in the prevention of muscle atrophy, osteoporosis and arthritis in the elderly. Beyond individual health benefits, physical activity is also linked to community wellbeing through the encouragement of social interaction.

In modern society, we generally take the relationship between physical activity and health as an unquestionable fact. Studies show that Australians are well aware of the benefits of regular exercise—just like we know smoking is bad and chocolate is a food to be enjoyed in moderation (Australian Institute of Health and Welfare 2018)! It is surprising, therefore, that the danger of an overly sedentary lifestyle was only proven empirically in the 1950s. It was at this time that epidemiologists recognised a relationship between a rise in diseases such as heart disease and a decrease in the need for incidental movement in daily life. Prior to this, for the majority of the population, the way people worked, travelled and accomplished other basic tasks of life was sufficiently active to maintain a healthy weight and level of fitness. Indeed, planned exercise was seen as an almost frivolous pursuit, rather than a critical component of a healthy lifestyle. This changed in the post-war era, when the decrease in incidental movement really gained pace. This was the era of technological progress, which, while entirely welcome, had the unintended consequence of 'engineering out' the need to move. Two English medical doctors—J.N. Morris and Margaret Crawford—set out to explore this concern by testing the hypothesis that sedentary workers suffered more heart disease than those in active jobs. Their study of early coronary heart disease in 3,800 corpses inspired the then ground-breaking claim that "men in physically-active jobs have a lower incidence of coronary (ischaemic) heart disease in middle age than men in physically-inactive jobs" (Morris and Crawford 1958, p. 5111). This is one of the first empirical studies to substantiate the now common knowledge that an absence of movement in daily life is unhealthy.

Physical Activity in Australia—How Are Australians Physically Active?

To provide an overview of the way Australians participate in physical activity, we first need to make a distinction between different types of activities. We divide physical activity into categories of recreational physical activity, organised sport and utilitarian physical activity. Table 4.1 provides a working definition and some popular Australian examples for each type of physical activity. It also contains examples of different built environment features associated with each form of activity. Of course, there are no firm rules around these categories. What we consider to be important in Australia is that, as a nation, we pride ourselves on a perceived legacy of success in organised sports. While this does not mean we are all avid participants in organised sport, it does have a subtle impact on the way we think about physical activity as individuals and the way our governments support different types of physical activity. For example, as a nation, and relative to other developed countries, government spending on elite sport is prioritised over other types of less organised physical activity (Australian Sports Commission 2015). Also, for many Australians, the idea of physical activity being linked to other activities of daily life—namely, transport—is

Table 4.1 Types of physical activity and supportive built environments

	Definition	Examples popular in Australia	Examples of supportive environments
Recreational Physical Activity	Physical activity that is planned, structured and purposive in the sense that improvement or maintenance of physical and/or mental health is the objective	Jogging Walking (through parks, bushwalking, dog-walking) Gym and gym classes Cycling and mountain biking Swimming Improvised play Golf	Private and outdoor gyms Private and public pools Public open spaces Dog parks Bushland areas and beaches Footpaths and cycleways Roads Linear parkways Golf courses Private backyards
Organised Sport	Physical activity that is planned and structured and, by its nature and organisation, is competitive and has an outcome	Competitive swimming/ running/cycling Cricket Football (rugby league and union) Soccer Netball Tennis Surf Life Saving	Outdoor and indoor sports facilities, including cricket pitches, netball, basketball and tennis courts; football and soccer fields; cycling velodromes; athletics tracks and swimming pools Stadiums Beaches
Utilitarian Physical Activity	Physical activity undertaken as part of day-to-day activity, physical activity that is associated with a specific purpose other than to be active; also referred to as Incidental Physical Activity	Active transport Taking the stairs Gardening Housework/ cleaning Physically active employment (most trades, nurses, cleaners, teachers)	Anywhere and everywhere we live, work and play! In particular: Footpaths and cycleways Roads End-of-trip facilities, such as bike racks, showers and changing-rooms Private and community gardens

relatively novel. Both of these subtle idiosyncrasies are reflected in the way we are physically active.

The Australian guidelines for a healthy amount of physical activity require <u>regular</u> participation and also specify target durations of time. These guidelines are outlined in Box 4.1. Statistics collected by the

Australian Institute of Health and Welfare (AIHW) indicate that many Australians struggle to adhere to the regularity and duration required by recommended guidelines (see Figure 4.1). In 2014–2015, just less than half (48%) of Australians aged 18–64 participated in sufficient physical activity per week (AIHW 2018). Overall, a higher proportion of women (58%) than men (53%) do not meet physical activity guidelines, and physical inactivity increases with age. For those aged 18–24, 42% of men and 51% of women do not meet physical activity guidelines. For those aged 75 and over, 67% of men and 81% of women do not meet physical activity guidelines. Perhaps most disturbing of all is that in 2014–2015, 80% of Australia's children aged 5–17 did not meet physical activity guidelines (Jongenelis et al. 2018).

Box 4.1   The Australian Physical Activity Guidelines

The Australian Physical Activity Guidelines recommend that healthy adults:

- Be active on most (preferably all) days each week
- Accumulate two and a half to five hours of moderate intensity physical activity or 75 to 150 minutes of vigorous intensity physical activity or an equivalent combination of both moderate and vigorous activities each week
- Do muscle strengthening activities at least two days each week
- Break up long periods of sitting as often as possible

There are separate guidelines for children and young people, and these generally advocate that children be more physically active, accumulating on average 60 minutes of activity per day. There are also guidelines for people over the age of 65, which encourage older people to continue enjoying 30 minutes of physical activity on most days. We recommend the guidelines advise that the amount of physical activity performed by an individual must be tailored to his or her physical and mental health.

Source: Adapted from AIHW 2018

With regard to utilitarian physical activity, it is difficult to find generalisable quantitative data on the way Australians are physically active through, for example, vigorous housework or gardening. It is also difficult to quantify participation in more active employment because the

Sufficiently active Australian
aged 18-64 for health benefits

48%

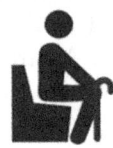
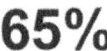

Inactive or insufficiently active
Australians aged 65+

65%

Inactive or insufficiently active
women aged 18-64

54%

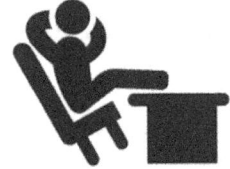

Inactive or insufficiently active
men aged 18-64

51%

Children and young people aged
5-17 who did not meet physical
activity recommendations

80%

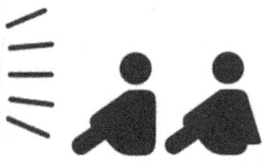

Children aged 5-8 who failed to
meet the physical activity
recommendations

64%

Figure 4.1 Australian participation in physical activity
Source: Adapted from AIHW 2018

amount of activity required to perform tasks varies greatly according to role and location. We do, however, have data on the use of active transport. Because this is a type of utilitarian physical activity very much impacted by how built environments are planned and managed, the way Australians participate in active transport is worthy of analysis.

The best indicator on the use of active transport in Australia is the journey to work (or commute) data from the Australian census. Regarding cycling, in 2016, rates ranged from just 2–5% of transport mode share for the commute across all urban areas. To compare, most cities in Northern and Western Europe have average commute cycling rates at least twice as high as those in Australia. The cycling cities of Copenhagen and Amsterdam average almost 50% (Bassett et al. 2008). While not yet represented in data on the journey to work, anecdotally there has been increased interest in cycling in Australia. Bikes have become attached to popular culture and are used to market everything from coffee to credit to (ironically) cars. Over 55% of Australian households own a bike. It seems, however, that while we like the idea of bikes, our propensity to actually ride for transport remains nascent. The Australian Bicycle Council and Austroads (Australia's peak organisation of road transport and traffic agencies) commission a National Cycling Participation Survey, which has been conducted every two years since 2011. The 2017 release of survey data showed declining rates of participation in cycling overall, and only 30% of riders were cycling for transport purposes (Australian Bicycle Council 2017). The good news is that cycling for transport is increasing in some inner urban areas in Australia's cities. In areas where densities are high, distances are short and an effort has been made to provide cycling infrastructure, the number of people cycling to work has increased markedly over the last 5–10 years. In Newtown, for example, a suburb in Sydney's gentrified Inner West, 4.9% of the population rode to work on the 2016 census day. In the inner Melbourne suburbs of Fitzroy North and Carlton North, cycling rates are as high as 15%. Yet in the suburbs—where the majority of people live—commuting to work by bike remains rare. Regarding walking to work, overall figures are similarly low, from 2.5% to 6.5%. These figures, however, mask even sharper variability between different localities. Again, in the inner urban areas of our major capital cities, walking captures are around 25–30% of the commute mode share.

How Can the Built Environment Support Physical Activity?

The built environment can be structured in ways to facilitate or constrain physical activity. The form of the built environment, incorporating residential and commercial density, land use mix, connectivity and accessibility, influences the way we move and what we do within that environment.

The way our urban areas are planned and managed— including the provision of open spaces, playgrounds and paths for walking and cycling— shapes the spaces where we are physically active for recreation. The built environment also shapes travel behaviour. This includes the desirability and practicality of walking and cycling for transport and the appeal of more sedentary options, such as private car use. The way the built environment shapes the time we spend on travel is also linked to the amount of leisure time available for other healthy pursuits, including recreational physical activity.

Motivating Australians To Be Physically Active

To understand the way the built environment supports physical activity in Australia, it helps to explore existing motivators and barriers to participation. Each year, the Australian Sports Commission collects data on participation in physical activity through the AusPlay national survey, which is a survey of over 20,000 Australians over the age of 15. It also incorporates interviews with over 4,000 parents/guardians of children aged 0–14.

In 2015–2016, the AusPlay survey found that for Australian adults up to middle age, time pressure is by far the main barrier to participating in physical activity. For older people, poor health or injury further inhibits participation. Barriers are different for children and harder to generalise. In part, this is due to the need to consider the schedules of both parent and child, as well as the preferences of both parties. The survey does show, however, that availability of transport, lack of time and cost are some of the key barriers to children's participation in organised sport in Australia (Australian Sports Commission 2016).

There is a series of Australian academic studies that has examined barriers to physical activity in more depth. For example, in 2010, Ester Cerin led a study at the University of Queensland examining perceived barriers to physical activity (Cerin et al. 2010). Using quantitative data from 2,194 Australian adults, the researchers found that lack of motivation was cited as a key barrier to all types of physical activity. In the context of comparing this study with the AusPlay survey mentioned above, we can see how things like lack of time may actually be a proxy for low motivation. Motivation is a very multifaceted concept, with several deep theoretical lineages, mainly based in psychology. To simplify this complexity and facilitate a brief analysis of the intersections between motivation, physical activity and built environments, we highlight three key requirements of motivation:

- We are in control of what we are doing (self-determination)
- We believe we can actually do it (perceived self-efficacy)
- We believe there is something in it for us (perceived benefit)

The way our urban areas are planned has both very direct and indirect links to all of these motivational factors, which we now explore.

Urban Planning, Self-Determination and Motivation to be Physically Active

Self-determination, in the context of physical activity, is an individual's ability to control whether he or she is physically active. Self-determination might be eroded by a physical inability to be active (for example, through disability, illness or injury) or by a very practical lack of time to be physically active (for example, if our spare time is taken up with work commitments, carer responsibilities or travel time). Clearly, there are times when physical activity is simply not possible, but if this occurs regularly, it could be argued that we are lacking in the self-determination component of motivation. Conceptualisation of self-determination as a key component of motivation exposes the way that it is not entirely within the control of the individual to be motivated, providing a hint as to why health programs based simply on individual behaviour change may be ineffective. Motivation is a product of our external circumstances as well as our individual will. For example, the way cities are planned influences the extent to which we have control over our time, including how much time is required to, for instance, travel to work or chauffeur children. Most Australian cities are spread out, with long distances between uses, and housing in our largest cities is increasingly unaffordable, leaving many destined to long periods of travel time. This is often not easily controlled on a day-to-day basis both because of its unpredictability and the fact that it is predetermined by where we live relative to the places we need to access for work, study, shopping or relaxation. As a result, Australia's dispersed cities and associated lengthy travel times potentially erode self-determination and therefore motivation for physical activity. Firstly, they ensure we are more likely to be time-poor and therefore must sacrifice activities not immediately demanding of our attention. Secondly, they detract from a sense that we are <u>in control</u> of what we do with our time. This lack of control is echoed through many domains of Australians' lives, including the increasing precariousness of employment and the insecurity of housing tenure. In short, it is very easy to paint a picture of an Australian society increasingly lacking tangible experiences of self-determination. This pervasive sense of not being in control of how we spend our time weakens motivation for activities that we believe to be discretionary. Unfortunately, this includes physical activity.

Urban Planning, Perceived Self-Efficacy and Motivation to be Physically Active

Perceived self-efficacy is the belief in one's ability to accomplish a task. In the context of physical activity, motivation may be low because we simply do not believe we have the ability to exercise appropriately. This component of physical activity was recently explored by a team from Western Australia's Curtin University. Led by clinical psychologist Michelle Jongenelis, the researchers asked 2,911 Australian adolescents between the ages of 12 and 17 what their key barriers to exercising were (Jongenelis et al. 2018). The answer 'I am not very good at physical activity' was a prevailing response. This suggests an inherent self-doubt in ability, and it is easy to see how finding an activity difficult, or not enjoyable, can erode motivation. Other reasons might include having tried and failed in the past, not knowing how much exercise to undertake or belief that the necessary facilities are unavailable for one's preferred exercise type. In the Australian context, it may be that our adoration of professional athletes and their super-human accomplishments actually works to highlight this perceived inability to do physical activity. The omnipresence of elite sport in Australian culture may well be detracting from our belief in ourselves and the value of practising a more moderate (and indeed healthier) exercise routine.

Urban planning can increase self-efficacy for physical activity by making it easy for people to exercise. The majority of the second section of this chapter is dedicated to how good urban planning can make physical activity an easy and obvious thing to do. We cover things such as ensuring equitable access to the spaces and streets that host exercise. We also discuss the need to make these provisions attractive, safe and logical so that people feel comfortable and welcomed. What is important here is that making things easy is not just about providing an attractive environment for the activity. It is also about boosting people's confidence in their ability to participate in regular exercise.

Urban Planning, Perceived Benefit and Motivation to be Physically Active

The final component of motivation is the perceived benefit derived from an activity. This is moderated by many things, most of which are intrinsic to the individual. Most people will feel that an activity has more benefits if it is undertaken in an attractive and safe place. The way built environments are planned and managed, therefore, has a role to play in enhancing perceived benefit from physical activity (and therefore motivation) by providing ample safe and well-maintained places for people to be active. For example, a 30-year-old woman in an outer suburb of Brisbane would like to use one of the many fitness apps available to do her own 20-minute stretching session outdoors most mornings. She plans to walk five minutes to the nearest park to do this. If the park closest to her home is attractive, green and well-kept, and she feels safe there, her experience of the session will be enhanced, reinforcing her motivation to continue the routine. Alternatively, if the park is vandalised, fronts a noisy major road and is sparsely furnished and planted, her experience of the undertaking will be undermined. She will perceive that the practice has less benefit to her, and her motivation to continue will be reduced. In short, if we have attractive places to go to exercise, the benefit we get from the activity is enhanced, and as a result, motivation increases. Again, this is about understanding some of the less direct and often unacknowledged reasons <u>why</u> the elements of a healthy built environment are so important.

This brief discussion of motivation highlights the fact that healthy built environments cannot just address the practical and environmental barriers to physical activity. Built environments are also deeply implicated in some of the more individual barriers, such as time availability and motivation. The remainder of this chapter concentrates on the broader elements of what makes an urban area supportive of physical activity. We first look at ways Australia's planning can support utilitarian physical activity, with a focus on encouraging walking and cycling. We then progress to ways urban planners are creating supportive environments specifically for recreational physical activity.

Planning for Utilitarian Physical Activity

Our analysis of barriers to physical activity highlights the importance of time and motivation. These barriers can both be overcome if physical activity is incorporated into other activities in our day-to-day lives. As outlined earlier in this chapter, we call this 'utilitarian physical activity'. Active transport is one of the most effective and well-researched types of utilitarian physical activity. Everyone needs to get from one place to another, and if we can do that in a physically active way, there is a dual benefit—physical activity for health and transportation for mobility. The achievement of these two outcomes, particularly when time is constrained, may well enhance motivation to be physically active.

The term 'active transport' is principally used in healthy built environment research and practice to imply walking and cycling for transport. Some studies also consider public transport to be active transport because the accessing and egressing of public transport inevitably require an active component (such as walking or cycling to the bus, train or tram stop). More contemporary studies, particularly those looking at children's active transport, also consider foot and kick scooters as active transport. For the purposes of this book, when we talk about active transport, we generally mean walking and cycling. If public transport is to be included in that mix, we mention it specifically. Often, active transport is contrasted with private car use, with the features of built environments to discourage private car use proposed as those that encourage active transport (Kent 2014). Sometimes, this is true. However, like so many elements of healthy built environments, it is never that simple (see

Box 9.1 in Chapter 9—Transport, Access and Health). So, how can good urban planning promote active transport as a physical activity?

Transport and Land Use for Active Transport: the Ds

Land use features associated with walking and cycling can be usefully categorised into five 'Ds'. The original 'three Ds', devised by Cervero and Kockelman (1997), are density, diversity and design, followed later by destination accessibility and distance (Ewing and Cervero 2001; Ewing and Cervero 2010). The influence of the Ds on active transport behaviour has been tested many times over and in numerous contexts. For example, a team at the University of Melbourne analysed data from 16,890 Victorian adults to demonstrate that higher densities, mixed uses and plentiful destinations are associated with more active transport and less car use (Badland et al. 2017). Research confirms that active transport is rarely supported through the provision of one D alone. Instead, a carefully tailored mix that is maintained over time is an absolute prerequisite. Table 4.2 describes each D principle. We then proceed to explore ways the D principles work together.

At the heart of the D principles is distance. The distance we are willing to walk or cycle is determined by a complex fusion of physical ability, the built environment, the amount of time and energy available for travel and physical activity and the desire to get from one place to another. With regard to cycling, Krizek et al. (2009) indicate high participation in bicycling trips of less than two and a half kilometres. Other studies show that people will cycle up to ten kilometres to access high-frequency public transport services (as reviewed by Pucher et al. 2010). Again, the best measure of the distance Australians are willing to cycle for transport is the Australian census, which records data on the way Australians travel to work. Recent analyses show that we have similar preferences to those cited in the international literature. For example, two-thirds of cycling journeys to work in Melbourne are approximately five kilometres or less, with 80% less than seven kilometres (Loader 2018). For walking, 400–500 metres (or around five minutes' duration) is generally accepted as a comfortable distance for most people. However, similar to cycling, various studies have shown that people will walk greater distances to access desirable destinations such as public transport hubs or other services (Besser and Dannenberg 2005). Using the South East Queensland Travel Survey, which involved 10,931 respondents, Burke and Brown (2007) present detailed information on the distances people walk for transport purposes in Brisbane. They report that the median distance people walk from home to all other places—using the walk mode only—is just under one and a half kilometres. In summary, all of this research suggests that the more desirable the destination, the further people are willing to walk or cycle to access it.

Table 4.2 The basics of the D principles for active transport

D principle	Description
Distance	Distance is usually expressed as distance to public transport. Because of the importance of distance as a barrier to active transport in low-density cities, we broaden this to refer to the expanse of space between all types of destinations. The distance people are willing to walk and cycle is a lot less than the distance that can be covered by a car in the same time. As a result, to promote walking and cycling in Australia's low-density, car-oriented cities, we need to reduce travel distances by bringing different uses closer together.
Density	Density is the degree of concentration of a variable of interest within a given urban area. The variable of interest might be population, residential dwelling units, employment, building floor area or something else. Active transport is generally encouraged by higher densities, but density in isolation will not encourage walking and cycling for transport.
Design	Design includes the layout of the street network and infrastructural elements that make a place safe and inviting. Street networks vary from dense urban grids of highly interconnected and straight streets to sparse suburban networks of curving streets with disconnected cul-de-sacs. The way walking and cycling paths are laid down and maintained, the design and adornment of streetscapes with green and natural features and the location and upkeep of infrastructure, such as seating, lighting, bike racks and signage, are important details that make an active transport journey achievable and enjoyable.
Diversity	Diversity is the relative variety of land uses in an urban area—for example, the mixing of residential, commercial and industrial uses. Areas with more diverse uses encourage active transport because they increase the likelihood that the things we need to access are within walking or cycling distance. Diversity can also add interest to an urban area, making it more attractive for those travelling at a slower pace.
Destinations	Destination accessibility measures ease of access to trip attractions. It may be regional or local. In some studies, it is the number of jobs or other attractions reachable within a given travel time and tends to be highest at central locations and lowest at peripheral ones.

To see a serious uptake of active transport in Australia, we need to bring commonly accessed uses closer together than they currently are. Australian cities are designed to accommodate private car use, and because cars travel so much faster than pedestrians or cyclists, the distances between uses in our cities are greater than in most European cities. To increase walking and cycling in Australia, we must reduce the distance people have to travel to access the things they regularly need. The key planning tools required to do this are increased densities (of residential, commercial and other uses) and increased diversity of uses (also known as mixed uses). Diversity of uses then enables strategic placement of destinations (including the places where we work and services such as shops and community facilities), making walking and cycling a possible and desirable option for more people. Chapter 9—Transport, Access and Health—outlines the ways densities can be increased, uses mixed and destinations strategically distributed in existing Australian urban areas to encourage active transport. We also discuss some of the complications associated with increased density in the introduction to Part III—Domains of the Built Environment.

Once distances are reduced by increased density, diversity and destinations, there is a need to focus on the design elements that make walking and cycling enjoyable, safe and an obvious transport option. The first step is to define a walking and cycling network at different scales—from the neighbourhood to the suburb and beyond. This network should be as direct as is safely possible, linking commonly accessed destinations such as shops, services, schools and public transport hubs. It should be continuous and uniform, crossing borders such as busy roads, suburb boundaries and Local government areas seamlessly. The detailed finishing elements of design should then be a priority, as these are just as important as increasing density and mixing uses within an area. A cracked footpath, misplaced light pole that intercepts a bike way or unkempt stretch of vacant blocks can be the difference between a neighbourhood where walking and cycling are pleasant and safe and one in which these are frustrating activities.

There have been many studies undertaken—and many words written—on the exact parameters of active transport network design and ways to implement the D principles. We urge some caution around the prescription of specific controls for walking and cycling environments, which is why we do not list any here. One of the key healthy planning principles is recognition that context is key and what works in one area may be unsuitable for another (see Chapter 11—Reflections on Principles of Healthy Planning). If detailed design advice is required, the Austroads *Guide to Traffic Management* contains basic details on ways to plan routes and infrastructure for cycling and walking. This is an extremely comprehensive and detailed guide, containing 13 modules covering everything from the design of a stop sign to the width of a freeway lane. They have also published a useful report called *Cycling Aspects of Austroads Guides*, which covers all of the cycling elements of the Austroads guide. There is an additional Austroads guide titled *Pedestrian-Cyclist Conflict Minimisation on Shared Paths and Footpaths*. All of these guides can be accessed free of charge from the Austroads website—www.austroads. com.au. Most Australian States and Territories have supplementary technical manuals for the planning and design of cycling and walking networks. In Appendix Two, we provide information on several excellent design guidelines.

In addition to the right mix of D principles, there are other things that urban planning can do to prioritise walking and cycling over other less healthy modes of transport (namely, the private car). Sometimes this is referred to as the sixth D because it is about managing the demand for private car use, often termed 'travel demand management'. The built environment can be modified to decrease demand for travel in many ways. Regulating car parking is a particularly effective mechanism. Limiting on-street car parking and placing strict controls on the amount of car parking available at both residential and commercial premises can have a significant impact on private car use, and even ownership, freeing up space for cycling and walking.

Finally, to encourage active transport, planners need to acknowledge that barriers are not only about time, cost, safety and motivation. Woven through the practicalities of travelling by bike or on foot are cultural attitudes. These can impede even the contemplation of cycling or walking for transport. In Australia, this is particularly relevant to cycling. At the heart of cycling cultures is contestation over road space, making safety a concern for existing cyclists and a barrier to the uptake of cycling. These issues are further explored in Box 4.2.

Box 4.2   Cycling safety and cultures

Cycling has a chequered history in Australia. Prior to the rise in popularity of the private car, it was relatively common to ride for transport. The use of bikes for transport decreased, however, as the distances between uses became longer and the car came to dominate roads. Today, it is an issue that polarises not only Australian roads but also Australian society. There is undoubtedly a resurgence of 'cycling cultures' in Australia. In the major cities, bikes have come to be associated with an ideal of inner urban living, where the café is just a quick ride away and it's entirely acceptable, quite possibly applauded, to arrive at the local pub or a friend's place on a bike. Outside of the inner cities, however, there is plenty of evidence to suggest that cycling and, in particular, cyclists are not universally accepted as legitimate users of road space. In an analysis of 326 newspaper articles published by the Australian press between 1998 and 2008, University of Sydney health promotion expert and avid cyclist, Chris Rissel, found that while a majority (60%) of articles reported cycling in a positive way, in most cases, positive representations discussed cycling as a practice, rather than cyclists per se.

Negative reports were more likely to feature discussions of cyclist behaviour (Rissel et al. 2010). Modern Australia has grown up during the era of the private car, and for most, daily life, the surrounding environment and attitudes are structured around access to private car use. Cyclists on our roads, and even those using the often inadequate infrastructure that is separated from the road, are regularly positioned as 'the other'. Cyclists are seen as belonging to a subordinate and somehow inferior group of road users.

Negative attitudes towards cyclists undoubtedly contribute to perceptions that cycling is an unsafe way to be physically active or travel. Concern for safety is a major barrier to the uptake of cycling in Australia (Bauman et al. 2008), and in many cases this perception is justified. For example, in an analysis of 2,847 nonfatal major trauma cases and 614 deaths from sport-related major trauma, cycling was the sport associated with the highest rates of trauma and death. This same study identified that these rates are increasing (Ekegren et al. 2018). Harassment from motorists adds to the perception that cycling is unsafe. Pre-empting this, health promotion specialist Kristiann Heesch from the Queensland University of Technology led a team to assess the incidence of harassment experienced by 1,830 Australian cyclists. They found that 76% of men and 72% of women had experienced harassment from people in cars over the previous 12 months. The most reported forms of harassment were driving too closely (66%), shouting abuse (63%) and making obscene gestures/sexual harassment (45%) (Heesch et al. 2011).

The passing of mandatory bicycle helmet laws in 1991 signalled a new focus on the safety of cyclists in Australia. These laws state that anyone on a bike must wear a helmet, and this rule is enforced by police. Upon its introduction, the legislation increased helmet use from about 30% to 80%. Unfortunately, this was coupled with a 40% decline in the number of people cycling (Rissel and Wen 2011). Possible barriers include the cost of the helmet and the need to store it somewhere at the end of the trip. Other barriers are the physical discomfort of wearing a helmet, particularly through Australia's hot summers. And finally, there is the issue of 'helmet hair'. Australian research has shown that both men and women have little desire to arrive at their destination with the sweaty imprint of their helmet ruining their hairstyle and betraying their mode of transport (Daley and Rissel 2011). This has caused some Australian researchers to argue that while helmets offer protection, they also discourage people from cycling (Rissel and Wen 2011). Others have countered this line of thinking, suggesting that helmets have been effective in reducing head injuries in collisions involving cycling (Olivier et al. 2016). At the time of writing, this informative and rich debate continues.

Addressing the tensions between drivers and cyclists will take both changes to the built environment and changes to attitudes and practices of driving cars and riding bikes. With regard to the built environment, separated facilities are by far the gold standard intervention. There is some research (principally pioneered by American engineer John Forester) indicating that separating cyclists from motorists ensures that car drivers are unfamiliar with how to pass a cyclist when they do inevitably meet (Forester 1993). In Australia, however, where cycling needs to be nurtured, an obvious demarcation—and preferably separation—between road users is vital. Concurrent with built environment interventions, we also need to focus on changing the attitudes of road users—both cyclists and car drivers. Australian roads need to be places where all legal users are recognised as legitimate. The Amy Gillett Foundation aims to do just that. This Australian foundation was established in 2005 following the death of Amy Gillett, who was tragically killed by a car driver while cycling in Germany with the Australian women's cycling team. The foundation, funded through donations, charity rides and corporate sponsorship, has led multiple initiatives to improve safety. One of their most visible and effective campaigns has been 'A Metre Matters'. This is a national campaign to legislate that when overtaking a bicycle, drivers must allow a minimum distance of a) one metre when the speed limit is 60 kilometres per hour or less and b) 1.5 metres when the speed limit is more than 60 kilometres per hour. Since launching the campaign in 2009, all States and Territories have either legislated or are trialling this new regulation.

Rebuilding Physical Activity Into Everyday Life

Built environments can be modified to encourage utilitarian physical activity well beyond the traditional focus on active transport. The places where we work have become a particular focus. We discuss the way urban planning in Australia can promote healthy workplaces in Chapter 10—Commercial, Service and Employment Spaces. Here, we focus on an intervention designed to encourage a more physically active approach to the traditional office job—the installation of sit-stand desks. While this is more in the realm of interior design and architecture than urban planning, the increasing popularity of sit-stand desks has sparked some interesting research that warrants mention here.

The phrase 'sitting is the new smoking' has become a popular axiom since it was coined in 2014 by Arizona-based Professor of Medicine, James Levine (who, incidentally, also invented the 'treadmill desk'). Swathes of offices around the world, including in Australia, have subsequently replaced their traditional desks with sit-stand contraptions. Employees are then urged to work standing, with some guidelines recommending standing for up to four hours every working day (see, for example, the consensus statement by Buckley et al. [2015], published in the *British Journal of Sports Medicine*). While it is undoubtedly true that prolonged sitting is bad for our health, studies are slowly emerging that question these original guidelines. In 2018, University of Sydney–based researcher, Josephine Chau, led an analysis of media reports of the so-called evils of sitting (Chau et al. 2017). Her research team discovered various interpretations of the guidelines. They also revealed a general failure to acknowledge that the empirical research used to back the four hours per day recommendation is questionable. Finally, Chau and her team exposed that those reporting and promoting the guidelines often had some affiliation with companies producing and marketing sit-stand desks. In summary, the tale of the sit-stand desk is a reminder of the need for moderation in built environment interventions to encourage physical activity. There are no magic bullets when it comes to allaying the health impacts of our less active modern lives. Change will surface only through a consistent, but balanced, approach, where a healthy amount of activity is enabled and encouraged rather than enforced and imposed.

Planning for Recreational Physical Activity

Although incorporating activity into everyday life has many benefits, the reality is that most Australians both perceive and practise physical activity as a recreational pursuit. The proper positioning and treatment of recreational spaces in our urban areas are therefore critical. In Chapter 8—Public Open Spaces—we provide specific information on designing and distributing healthy public open spaces. Here, we take some time to highlight some particularly Australian recreational physical activities and explore the environments that host them.

The Importance of Simply Having a Close-By Place

For most Australians, time availability makes it difficult to satisfy physical activity guidelines solely through competitive and organised sports. While sports facilities are an important piece of the puzzle, just as critical is ensuring that all Australians live within walkable distance of a green, outdoor and public 'place to go' to be active. This might be a place for impromptu play with children, somewhere to walk to or a place in which to stretch or exercise. Australia's planners are at the frontline of the provision and protection of public recreational spaces and uses in our cities. Public parks, gardens, walking trails, outdoor gyms, cycleways, ovals, off-leash dog parks and playing fields—these are the spaces in a city that make physical activity an easy and enjoyable part of daily life.

Our key concern with the way we plan and manage public open space in Australia is not necessarily the amount provided, although that is important. We are particularly interested in the way these places are fitted out and maintained. There are many studies across Australia that have quantified the amount of public open space available for recreation in Australian cities (for example, Astell-Burt et al. 2014). Less work has been done, however, to assess the quality of open space available. An exception is a study led by David Crawford as part of the 'Children Living in Active Neighbourhoods' study. Using data from 540 families in Melbourne, this research examined relationships between neighbourhood socio-economic status and features of public open spaces hypothesised to influence children's physical activity. It was concluded that, compared with public open space in lower socio-economic neighbourhoods, spaces in the highest socio-economic neighbourhoods had more amenities, such as picnic tables, trees providing shade, a water feature, walking and cycling paths, lighting and signage. There were no differences across neighbourhoods in the quantity of playgrounds or the number of recreational facilities (Crawford et al. 2008, 2010). This suggests that while many people in Australian urban areas do have walkable access to some kind of public open space, these spaces are not maintained consistently. To be motivated to do regular physical activity, people need spaces that are not only nearby but are also attractive and safe. Fine-grained research is required to explore the extent to which barriers to recreational physical activity are as much about upkeep and management of open spaces as they are about provision of the space.

Walking and Cycling for Recreation

Walking for recreation is the most popular type of planned recreational physical activity in Australia (Australian Sports Commission 2016). Cycling for recreation in Australia is also popular. In fact, over 80% of the Australians who ride a bike do so for recreation rather than transport (Australian Bicycle Council 2017). The environments that encourage utilitarian walking and cycling are not necessarily conducive to walking and cycling for recreation. Perceived and actual safety remain of primary importance, as does the provision of street networks that are legible and well maintained, with footpaths, shade and lighting. Aesthetics, however, replace destinations and network density, with recreational walkers not particularly interested in taking the most direct route. Indeed, research in Australia has found that the provision of special-purpose walking trails is more likely to encourage recreational walking (Sugiyama et al. 2015) and cycling (Badland 2017). This is possibly a reflection of our car-oriented society, where walking and cycling are not automatically considered transport options but are readily associated with recreational activities. Like public recreational facilities, walking and cycling trails for recreation are the domain of Local government authorities. These authorities can apply for grants from Federal and State bodies to fund improvements and maintenance of recreational facilities. A great example of a walking and cycling trail developed and funded collaboratively by Local and State government authorities is the GreenWay in Sydney, described in Box 4.3.

Box 4.3   The GreenWay in inner Sydney

The GreenWay, in the inner urban area of Sydney's west, is an exemplary piece of green infrastructure for healthy and environmentally sustainable living. It was originally an initiative involving four adjoining Local Councils, bringing Local government professionals from disparate disciplinary backgrounds together to work collaboratively with the community.

The GreenWay connects two of Sydney's most important waterways—the Parramatta and Cooks Rivers—via a 5-kilometre light rail, active transport and urban environmental corridor. It follows the route of a light-rail service (converted from the former freight rail line), integrating cycling, walking and public transport. It is a significant community hub for the arts and bushcare and connects to several recreational facilities, including outdoor gyms, sporting fields, children's playgrounds, a dog park with café and picnic areas.

The GreenWay serves as a local outdoor classroom, modelling urban sustainability for school and university students. An extensive educational program of resources developed for primary schools is now recommended as best practice for geography studies by the New South Wales Department of Education. Several universities use the GreenWay to run multidisciplinary classes involving students from the built environment and health. They research different aspects of the GreenWay, experiencing complex, real-world, urban sustainability and health issues in holistic and integrated ways. Over the last few years, students have put a raft of different issues under the microscope, making recommendations about light-rail accessibility, pedestrian safety, disabled access, lighting and shared walking and cycling paths.

The GreenWay demonstrates how green corridors, with shared cycling and walking paths, can encourage much more than just physical activity. Community members from different generations, socio-economic backgrounds and cultures are connected in an outdoor setting that is supportive of their physical and mental health.

See www.greenway.org.au/ for further information.

Conclusion

This chapter opened by proposing that the term 'physical activity' can be used to describe any type of human movement. Physical activity need not be planned or linked to a sport; it can just as easily be gardening, housework, walking to the bus or scooting to school. The key message is that to be healthy, a human body needs to be active, yet our environments have evolved to minimise the amount of physical effort needed to live a modern life. This minimisation can be seen in the facts: less than half of Australians participate in enough physical activity for health, and over 80% of children are not sufficiently active.

The chapter proceeded to explore some of the things that prevent Australians from being physically active and urban planning's role in overcoming these barriers. We concentrated on motivation, highlighting the need for all Australians to have adequate access to quality open spaces that are safe and well maintained. By drawing the link directly between motivation, time and broader city structure, we have unpacked some of the ways urban decision-making can, and does, influence the extent to which Australians are physically active.

We concluded by dipping into some of the vast literature that exists on designing urban areas for physical activity. Physical activity has been a key interest for healthy built environment professionals and academics in Australia and around the world. Relative to other health risk factors (including the other domains in this book), the link between urban planning and physical activity has informed more guidelines, checklists, interventions and journal articles. We have purposefully eschewed a comprehensive review of this body of work. This has enabled an exploration of some of the less obvious links between built environments and physical activity. We urge readers interested in more detailed design guidance for physical activity to review some of the documents detailed in Appendix Two. Again, we preface the use of these guidelines with the acknowledgement that context is key, as is the need to appreciate and understand the particular qualities and characteristics of each unique community and circumstance.

References

Astell-Burt, T., Feng, X., Mavoa, S., Badland, H. M. and Giles-Corti, B. (2014) Do low-income neighbourhoods have the least green space? A cross-sectional study of Australia's most populous cities. *BMC Public Health*, 14 p. 292.

Australian Bicycle Council (2017) *Australian Cycling Participation: Results of the 2017 National Cycling Participation Survey*, Austroads, Sydney, NSW.

Australian Institute of Health and Welfare (2018) *Behavioural Risk Factors: Physical Activity Overview*. AIHW, Canberrra, ACT.

Australian Sports Commission (2016) *AusPlay: Participation Data for the Sport Sector*, Australian Government, Canberra.

Badland, H., Mavoa, S., Boulangé, C., Eagleson, S., Gunn, L., Stewart, J., David, S. and Giles-Corti, B. (2017) Identifying, creating, and testing urban planning measures for transport walking: Findings from the Australian national liveability study. *Journal of Transport & Health*, 5 pp. 151–162.

Bassett Jr, D. R., Pucher, J., Buehler, R., Thompson, D. L. and Crouter, S. E. (2008) Walking, cycling, and obesity rates in Europe, North America and Australia. *Journal of Physical Activity and Health*, 5(6) pp. 795–814.

Bauman, A., Rissel, C., Garrard, J., Ker, I., Speidel, R. and Fishman, E. (2008) *Getting Australia Moving: Barriers, Facilitators and Interventions to Get More Australians Physically Active Through Cycling*, Cycling Promotion Fund, Melbourne.

Besser, L. M. and Dannenberg, A. L. (2005) Walking to public transit: Steps to help meet physical activity recommendations. *American Journal of Preventive Medicine*, 29(4) pp. 273–280.

Buckley, J. P., Hedge, A., Yates, T., Copeland, R. J., Loosemore, M., Hamer, M., Bradley, G. and Dunstan, D. W. (2015) The sedentary office: An expert statement on the growing case for change towards better health and productivity. *British Journal of Sports Medicine*, 49(21) pp. 1357–1362.

Burke, M. and Brown, A. (2007a) Active Transport in Brisbane: How Much Is Happening and What Are Its Characteristics? in *Proceedings of the State of Australian Cities National Conference, Adelaide, South Australia*, University of South Australia, Adelaide, pp. 656–667.

Cerin, E., Leslie, E., Sugiyama, T. and Owen, N. (2010) Perceived barriers to leisure-time physical activity in adults: An ecological perspective. *Journal of Physical Activity and Health*, 7(4) pp. 451–459.

Cervero, R. and Kockelman, K. (1997) Travel demand and the 3Ds: Density, diversity, and design. *Transportation Research Part D: Transport and Environment*, 2(3) pp. 199–219.

Chau, J. Y., Mcgill, B., Freeman, B., Bonfiglioli, C. and Bauman, A. (2017) Overselling Sit-Stand Desks: News Coverage of Workplace Sitting Guidelines. *Health Communication* pp. 1–7.

Crawford, D., Cleland, V., Timperio, A., Salmon, J., Andrianopoulos, N., Roberts, R., Giles-Corti, B., Baur, L. and Ball, K. (2010) The longitudinal influence of home and neighbourhood environments on children's body mass index and physical activity over 5 years: The CLAN study. *International Journal of Obesity*, 34(7) pp. 1177–1187.

Crawford, D., Timperio, A., Giles-Corti, B., Ball, K., Hume, C., Roberts, R., Andrianopoulos, N. and Salmon, J. (2008) Do features of public open spaces vary according to neighbourhood socio-economic status? *Health and Place*, 14(4) pp. 889–893.

Daley, M. and Rissel, C. (2011) Perspectives and images of cycling as a barrier or facilitator of cycling. *Transport Policy*, 18(1) pp. 211–216.

Ekegren, C. L., Beck, B., Simpson, P. M. and Gabbe, B. J. (2018) Ten-year incidence of sport and recreation Injuries resulting in major trauma or death in Victoria, Australia, 2005–2015. *Orthopaedic Journal of Sports Medicine*, 6(3). doi:10.1177/2325967118757502

Ewing, R. and Cervero, R. (2001) Travel and the built environment: A synthesis. *Transportation Research Record*, 1780 pp. 87–114.

Ewing, R. and Cervero, R. (2010) Travel and the built environment: A meta-analysis. *Journal of the American Planning Association*, 76(3) pp. 265–294.

Forester, J. (1993) *Effective Cycling*, MIT Press, Cambridge, MA.

Heesch, K. C., Garrard, J. and Sahlqvist, S. (2011) Incidence, severity and correlates of bicycling injuries in a sample of cyclists in Queensland, Australia. *Accident Analysis and Prevention*, 43(6) pp. 2085–2092.

Jongenelis, M. I., Scully, M., Morley, B., Pratt, I. S. and Slevin, T. (2018) Physical activity and screen-based recreation: Prevalences and trends over time among adolescents and barriers to recommended engagement. *Preventive Medicine*, 106 pp. 66–72.

Kent, J. L. (2014) Carsharing as active transport: What are the potential health benefits? *Journal of Transport & Health*, 1(1) pp. 54–62.

Krizek, K., Forsyth, A. and Baum, A. (2009) *Walking and Cycling International Literature Review*, Department of Transport, Melbourne, Victoria.

Loader, C. (2018) *What Does the Census Tell Us About Cycling to Work?* https:// chartingtransport.com/2014/01/27/census-cycling-to-work/ [Accessed 28 May 2018].

Morris, J. N. and Crawford, M. D. (1958) Coronary heart disease and physical activity of work. *British Medical Journal*, 2(5111) pp. 1485–1496.

Olivier, J., Boufous, S. and Grzebieta, R. H. (2016) No strong evidence bicycle helmet legislation deters cycling: A focus on helmet legislation detracts from concerns about cycling infrastructure and safety. *Medical Journal of Australia*, 205(2) pp. 54–55.

Pucher, J., Dill, J. and Handy, S. (2010) Infrastructure, programs, and policies to increase bicycling: An international review. *Preventive Medicine*, 50 (Suppl. 1) pp. S106–S125.

Rissel, C., Bonfiglioli, C., Emilsen, A. and Smith, B. J. (2010) Representations of cycling in metropolitan newspapers–changes over time and differences between Sydney and Melbourne, Australia. *BMC Public Health*, 10 p. 371.

Rissel, C. and Wen, L. M. (2011) The possible effect on frequency of cycling if mandatory bicycle helmet legislation was repealed in Sydney, Australia: A cross sectional survey. *Health Promotion Journal of Australia*, 22(3) pp. 178–183.

Sugiyama, T., Shibata, A., Koohsari, M. J., Tanamas, S. K., Oka, K., Salmon, J., Dunstan, D. W. and Owen, N. (2015) Neighborhood environmental attributes and adults' maintenance of regular walking. *Medicine and Science in Sports and Exercise*, 47(6) pp. 1204–1210.

5 Planning for Social Interaction

Introduction: Why Is Social Interaction Important for Health?

A sense of support, community and belonging within the places where people live, work and travel is an influential determinant of mental and physical health. Indeed, internationally well-regarded psychologist, Roger S. Ulrich, once proclaimed that "low social support may be as great a risk factor in mortality as cigarette smoking" (Ulrich 1999, p. 42). Belonging fosters perceptions of security, confidence and comfort, which can encourage people to be physically active in their neighbourhood as well as socially connected to others.

At the heart of notions such as community, belonging and connection are social interactions. Interactions with other people are the fundamental basis of what it means for us to be social beings. They are an innate biological need with both psychological and physical health consequences. Without interaction, the regulation of cellular processes deep within the body is disrupted, predisposing us to premature ageing and, ultimately, premature mortality. This makes sense when we consider that early in our history as a species, we survived and prospered only by banding together—in couples, families and tribes. Interaction was a way to ensure mutual protection and assistance. The pain of isolation, therefore, evolved like any other form of pain—a way to protect us from harm. Too much social isolation feels unpleasant because it is a signal that connections to others are weak and need to be repaired (Cacioppo et al. 2011).

Social Interaction in Australia

In an age where technological developments have meant that it has never been easier to reach out and contact someone, many Australians feel lonely and isolated. They have no one to confide in or assist them, and they lack the friendships and social connections they desire.

(Flood 2005, p. 36)

How and Why Do We Interact?

The above quote is from the conclusion to a report commissioned by the national think tank The Australia Institute titled *Mapping Loneliness in Australia*. While the report analyses data from 2005, its key conclusions remain contemporary and are supported by more recent data from the General Social Survey. Conducted every four years by the Australian Bureau of Statistics (ABS), this survey includes measures of social and civic participation, interactions with others and the degree of control people feel they have over issues of importance. The most recent General Social Survey, conducted in 2014, contains data from 12,932 Australians aged 15 years and older. It shows decreased participation in social groups, such as those focused on sport or recreation, arts or heritage and religious or spiritual associations. It also indicated that Australians were less likely in 2014 to be involved in civic and political groups than they were in 2010. The good news is that the number and variety of attachments people reported were high. Nearly everyone (95%) surveyed in 2014 felt able to get support from outside their household in a time of crisis. However, the likelihood of seeking that support from a neighbour (as opposed to a friend, relative or colleague) is in decline. This indicates that the way Australians nurture attachments through day-to-day interactions is changing.

Box 5.1   Clubs in Australia

Organised clubs have traditionally played an important role in shaping and sustaining Australian communities. Throughout the 19th and 20th Centuries, clubs were a conduit for bridging the distance between city and country typical of the Australian landscape. They have provided a structure around which subsets of community groups can unite. The website clubsofaustralia.com. au claims to host data of over 36,000 clubs across the nation. The list on this site covers clubs from literally A-Z and includes sporting, book, chess and photography clubs as well as everything in between. Australia has a particularly rich history of participation in international service clubs such as Rotary and Lions. Apex is a similar service club organisation that is unique to Australia. Although membership in these clubs has followed the general trend and is in slow decline, service clubs remain important forums for community participation and charity work, particularly in regional and rural areas.

At the pinnacle of the clubs' hierarchy in Australia are those that are licensed and registered. These are not-for-profit, member-based organisations, differentiated from other clubs based on their having an actual premises and a liquor and/or gaming license, which is issued by the State government. Many of these clubs make a lot of money from betting and gaming (in particular, poker machines). Although this money is filtered back into the community through club activities and maintenance of the club venue, the registered clubs' association has been accused of supporting gambling addiction and being over-reliant on gambling as an income source. Nevertheless, registered clubs maintain that their central objective is to provide infrastructure and services for the community. Reflecting this, they are usually associated with a core purpose, such as the promotion of sporting activities (for example, a rugby league club) or veterans' welfare (for example, the Returned Services League [RSL]). At the time of writing, there were over 6,000 registered clubs in Australia, made up of bowling clubs (24%), sporting and recreation clubs (24%), golf clubs (17%), RSLs (15%), community and workers' clubs (4%) and cultural and religious clubs (4%). In terms of supporting a strong, interactive community, the main contribution of registered clubs is that they are the primary source of funding for many of the 36,000 community groups mentioned above. This might be through financial sponsorship or the provision of facilities, such as a room in which to meet.

It is worth noting that while participation in clubs is generally enjoyed equally by both women and men, there are still about 30 single-sex clubs dotted around our capital cities, the majority of which are male-only (often known as 'gentlemen's clubs'). The oldest of these is Sydney's The Australian Club, founded in 1838. These clubs originally provided a way for early pioneer farmers from the regions to maintain city contacts. Today, men continue to go to these clubs to escape city life and bond with friends. It could be argued that this is ostensibly a healthy practice. But, as celebrated Australian journalist Malcolm Knox puts it, "It's just a bit weird that half of the human race—wives, mothers, daughters, sisters, friends—can be seen as part of 'the strain of modern life' " (Knox 2009).

Lonely or Just Alone?

The absence of regular contact with others, either those around us in the community or our family and friends, increases the risk of feeling socially disconnected—a feeling that is commonly termed 'loneliness'. Loneliness, however, is not necessarily a result of being alone (Franklin and Tranter

2011). We can be surrounded by people, yet still feel isolated. This high-lights the fact that the way people experience loneliness is subjective, making it a difficult concept for researchers to measure. In Australia, the best source of quantitative data on loneliness comes from the longitudinal Household Income and Labour Dynamics in Australia (HILDA) study. Using this data, another report by The Australia Institute found that one in three Australians experienced an episode of loneliness between 2001 and 2009. Forty percent of these people experienced more than one epi-sode. People living in lone-person and lone-parent households were, on average, almost twice as likely to experience loneliness. There were also gender-based differences, with men more likely to be lonely compared with women, and adult males in their mid-20s to mid-40s the most lonely (Baker 2012). The findings in this report contradict the broader societal view in Australia that loneliness is predominantly a state or emotion expe-rienced by the elderly. Indeed, there is strong evidence to suggest that the majority of people in Australia aged 65 and older are neither lonely nor socially isolated (Aged and Community Services Australia 2015). These results are clarified by Flood's aforementioned review, which found that just 7% of older Australians reported experiences of loneliness—below the 9% average cited for the general population (Flood 2005). We cau-tion that these figures on older persons' experiences of isolation need to be viewed in the context that this population is more vulnerable to the negative impacts of loneliness than younger people. It is important, how-ever, to acknowledge that everyone is susceptible to loneliness.

To sum up this brief review of social interaction in Australia, the last two decades have witnessed changes in practices of connection and con-tact across the country. There is a general downward trend in the amount of face-to-face and incidental interactions we have and a shift towards more mediated interactions based on networks (either online or through an organised channel such as a school or workplace). This is a concern for sociologists (Grenade and Boldy 2008). If the only interactions we have are with the like-minded people we choose as our associates, we risk becoming blind to, and intolerant of, diversity—a process we discuss in detail below. This concern points to the fact that there are different types of interactions, with some more health-promoting than others. We now outline these different types as a prelude to exploring the most effective ways the built environment can support social interaction.

How Can the Built Environment Support Social Interaction?

A Hierarchy of Interactions

The quality and quantity of interactions required for optimal health are deeply personal and will be different for every individual. Research shows, however, that a variety of interactions is essential for wellbeing. This has been expressed in many ways in the literature, many of which can be traced to theories of psychological development, such as Maslow's hierarchy of needs, which places belonging as central to human flourishing. American-based neuroscientist John Cacioppo has written extensively on a lack of social interaction as a risk factor for poor health. He proposes a more minimal model of the types of interactions required for health based on three levels of connections:

> Level One: up-close and personal relationships, such as with a long-term partner
> Level Two: less intense but still regular connections between extended family and friends
> Level Three: interactions with the people who inhabit the neighbourhoods, workplaces and other spaces around us
> (Cacioppo et al. 2011)

The way Australia's urban areas are planned and managed can shape all three of these levels. For example, by providing jobs in close proximity to housing, planning can help reduce commute times, providing more opportunities for people to be at home with family (Level One). Planning also influences, to an extent, housing affordability, enabling family and friends to remain in close proximity (should they choose), rather than having to move away simply to afford a home (Level Two). These less direct impacts of urban form on social interaction are important. However, in this chapter, we focus specifically on Cacioppo's Level Three connection—incidental social interactions. This is in recognition of the many and varied ways Australian built environments can promote positive interactions within our immediate community.

The Importance of Incidental Interactions

We mentioned above that social interactions in modern Australian society are increasingly the result of existing networks. This simply means that, for many Australians, social interaction is linked to organised activities, including work, sport, a child's school and membership to a common interest group. Increasingly, these ties are both initiated and augmented online. As a result, they do not necessarily occur in the spaces where we physically spend our time. Incidental interactions are in between these formalised and networked connections. This is the day-to-day meeting and greeting of people who live, work and travel in the same spaces and at the same times as us. These interactions may not be with the people we would normally choose to associate with. Indeed, we may not even know them by name, nor speak to them for lengthy periods. Yet history, research and common sense all tell us that incidental interactions are critical components of the health of communities and individuals within those communities. They are small events that enrich connection to place, promote a duty of caring, increase perceptions of safety and belonging and decrease feelings of loneliness and isolation. It is through these incidental interactions that we learn to cooperate, tolerate and trust relative strangers. If the majority, or all, of our interactions with other people are with those we have met through a common interest or history, we risk becoming blind to diversity. Our ability to appreciate and respect difference is eroded. Furthermore, incidental interactions pave the way for more sustained interactions with those around us. They make it possible for more organised activities to flourish and are the first step in the establishment of enduring connections to people and place.

Incidental interactions thrive on regular contact. There is a scene in the iconic Australian movie Crocodile Dundee (1986) where Mick Dundee, a stereotypical outback Aussie bloke, walks down a very busy 5th Avenue in New York. He attempts to acknowledge every single person he passes with the classic Australian greeting 'G'day' but struggles with the relative onslaught of strangers and soon gives up. Although it makes for an amusing scene in a movie, outside of some small country towns, it would be unusual in Australia to simply say hello to a total stranger. This shifts, however, when we see that stranger more regularly. We start to realise that they share something in common with us—even if it is the 7.16 am train, the postcode where we live, the place where we buy our coffee or our morning walking routine. Regular chance meetings make it easier for us to say good morning, comment on the weather or simply just nod in greeting. And research unequivocally demonstrates that a community rich in these subtle interactions is more likely to be a healthy one (see, for example, Umberson and Montez 2010). These are the exchanges that give a space the potential to feel safe and welcoming, encouraging people to feel that they belong within it, living lives with coherency and connection.

Interaction and the Importance of Feeling Safe

Incidental interactions do not occur in spaces that feel unsafe. Following this logic, multiple studies have examined the links between crime rates and community and individual wellbeing. For example, a team led by Thomas Astell-Burt from Wollongong University used data from over 37,000 Australian participants in the 45 and Up Study to analyse links between crime rates and walking for recreation (Astell-Burt et al. 2016). Their quantitative analysis did not find a positive link between objectively measured crime rates and walking. Based on this result, they concluded that the link between crime and walking for recreation is questionable. This obviously counterintuitive finding indicates a dire need for studies such as this to incorporate perceived measures of crime, rather than actual rates of crime. It is not whether a place is deemed to be dangerous by crime statistics that will prevent social interactions. It is whether that place <u>feels</u> safe for those experiencing the interactions. Recognising this, there are many studies that do incorporate perceived safety into their analysis. Sarah Foster and a team from the University of Western Australia have published such a study using data from the landmark longitudinal RESIDE study. Their findings indicate a potential causal relationship between residents' perceptions of safety from crime and the uptake of recreational walking (Foster et al. 2016).

In assessing links between built environments and crime, planners often reference the concept of Crime Prevention Through Environmental Design (CPTED). CPTED has emerged over the last 30 years as the umbrella term for the design and construction of built form to reduce the incidence of crime and community fear of crime. The concept applies to crimes against public and private property (such as vandalism) and extends to crimes against the person (such as physical assault). What is known as first-generation CPTED is based on four key strategies:

1. 'Territoriality': encouraging a sense of ownership
2. 'Natural surveillance': encouraging eyes on the street
3. 'Activity support': encouraging use over vacancy
4. 'Access control': balancing surveillance and use with privacy

(Cozens et al. 2005)

When successfully adopted, these strategies have been shown to reduce opportunities to commit crime and increase all-important perceptions of safety. Although grounded in a long tradition of research and practice, the efficacy of first-generation CPTED in modern societies has recently been reassessed. Many of the critiques of first-generation CPTED relate to its over-reliance on structural adjustments and the inability of the planning system to implement solutions effectively. Research in New South Wales, for example, has uncovered substantial variations in the ways CPTED assessments are applied at the local level. This results in the assessment process proving ineffective in bringing about actual change to the built environment (Clancey 2011).

In recognition of some of the failings of first-generation CPTED, both researchers and practitioners have proposed that strong and connected communities are just as important in preventing crime and promoting safety as territoriality and eyes on the street. Indeed, CPTED pioneers Gregory Saville and Gerry Cleveland have advocated that instead of "neighbourhoods of watchers, we need a sense of community where people care about who they are watching" (Saville 2009, p. 389). This recognition has led to the emergence of what is known as second-generation CPTED. The four pillars of second-generation CPTED are as follows:

1. Social cohesion
2. Community connectivity
3. Community culture
4. Threshold capacity

(Cozens 2015)

Social cohesion is considered to be the mainstay, conceptualised by environmental criminologists as a community that is united in the protection of its local area. We propose that incidental interactions are a good catalyst for social cohesion. This is because such interactions promote an awareness of the steady state of neighbourhood life. If we are interacting with the people around us, we are compelled to notice when something looks, or even feels, amiss. Incidental interactions also promote a sense of caring and belonging—they are the beginnings of a sense of responsibility for the welfare of those around us. In this sense, the principles of second-generation CPTED become mutually reinforcing. Interactions promote a sense of safety, and a sense of safety promotes further interactions.

Nature Inspires Interaction

The bond between human beings and other living, natural systems is well researched. A healthy built environment simply must preserve and feature natural elements. These range from street trees and grassed verges to large tracts of bushland. They include companion and assistance animals and wildlife, such as birds and insects. Natural elements are important for interaction because they provide objects of fascination that become talking points. They also enliven spaces, making them more pleasurable places to traverse or linger in. In Chapter 8—Public Open Spaces—we discuss ways that natural elements can be planned into our cities and elaborate on the health benefits of the presence of greenery. Here, we focus on one specific conduit for interactions initiated by other-than-human elements—the keeping of companion animals.

Box 5.2   Companion and assistance animals

Our focus in this chapter is mostly on companion animals, but it is important to note that assistance animals also have close relationships with humans. For example, working animals, many of whom are dogs, perform a multitude of jobs, such as controlling livestock on farms, sniffing out illicit drugs or other contraband, searching for missing persons and guarding premises. Assistance animals—including guide dogs for the blind, hearing dogs for those with auditory limitations and therapy animals—also help people live independent and healthy lives.

Companion Animals in the City

In Australia, the best data on rates of companion animal ownership is collected by a consortium of veterinary pharmaceutical companies, Animal Medicines Australia. Their latest survey of over 2,000 Australians estimates that more than 24 million pets live in Australia today (Animal Medicines Australia 2016). This is slightly higher than the human population, which, in 2016, was 23.77 million! At 62%, Australia has one of the highest household rates of pet ownership in the world. Around 5.7 million of Australia's 9.2 million households are home to a pet, with many having more than one dog, cat, bird, fish, reptile or some other type of animal. Regarding popular types of pet, almost two in five households have one or more dogs (38%) while nearly three in ten households have one or more cats (29%). More than one in ten households also keep fish (12%), and a similar proportion of households are home to pet birds (12%).

There is a wealth of research exploring the idea that human-animal interactions can enhance human physical health and psychological wellbeing (see, for example, the review by Cutt et al. 2007). As many pet owners will testify, pets bring a unique experience of affection, enjoyment, companionship and distraction. Such anecdotes are supported by studies associating pet ownership with a diversity of therapeutic, psychological, physiological and psychosocial benefits. For example, companion animals have been linked to reduced severity of depression and anxiety as well as amelioration of bereavement. Pets have also been associated with reductions in cardiovascular disease risk factors, particularly high blood pressure. Although such research has focused predominantly on the benefits to individual pet owners, this work is complemented by a body of scholarship suggesting that pets can also generate broader social sustainability, which has benefits not only for individual owners but also the wider community (Wood et al. 2005). This includes the mitigating effects of animals on loneliness and social isolation. It also includes companion animal contributions to place-making by providing a talking point (Thompson 2016). Despite some discourse around the negative public and environmental health implications of pets (for example, the devastating impact of aggressive dog behaviour and the environmental damage associated with the hunting instincts of cats), the weight of evidence supports their health-enhancing potential.

With so much to gain from having companion animals in our lives, it is important that we provide supportive built environments for them. It is often urban planners who are charged with seeking ways to incorporate pets into modern lifestyles and communities. There are several ways planners and other built environment professionals in Australia are working to do this.

Firstly, we are seeking to ensure that people can care for companion animals in their homes. Many cities in Australia are experiencing densification, with more of our growing populations expected to call apartments home in the future. In Australia, Strata Title governs the majority of apartments and other forms of attached dwellings, such as townhouses. Strata Title allows for separate ownership of each apartment within a building and governance through a 'body corporate' consisting of property owners. Each State and Territory maintains its own strata laws, which are used to regulate matters relating to the use and maintenance of common property. These laws contain common rules, including those that regulate the keeping of companion animals. Until recently, the default position of these regulations was to prohibit the keeping of companion animals except in circumstances where body corporate permission was obtained. We have seen a shift across the country, however, with many States rescinding restrictive blanket prohibitions. For example, in New South Wales, the default position of a body corporate, prior to 2016, was that 'an owner or occupier of a lot may keep an animal on the lot or the common property *with the written approval* of the owners' corporation'. In 2016, this was amended to read that 'an owner or occupier of a lot may keep an animal on the lot, *if the owner or occupier gives the owners' corporation written notice* that it is being kept on the lot'. While this is a vast improvement, the law does not necessarily apply to titles registered prior to 1996. As a result, there are still many apartment buildings that deny owners and tenants the right to keep a companion animal. This becomes even more complex for people renting apartments. Again, in New South Wales, the tenancy law has a standard agreement that offers landlords two choices: to disallow all companion animals from being kept on the premises or to authorise the keeping of a specified companion animal or animals. While these statements can be erased manually as needed, the default position is usually 'no pets allowed' (Power 2016).

To realise the full potential of companion animals to foster interactions, we also need to provide spaces in the public realm where owners are able to be with their pets. Dogs are the main domesticated animals to traverse public spaces with their owners. Australia's high rates of dog ownership are reflected in the increasing propensity for people to be out and about with their dogs. This may take the form of dog-walking in the street or trips to a dog park, dog-friendly beach, café, pub or other recreational area. There is strong evidence that a well-behaved dog in a public space is a conduit for exactly the type of incidental social interactions that are the focus of this chapter. These interactions have been explored in detail by Lisa Wood of the University of Western Australia, whose research demonstrates the way the benefits of companion animal ownership ripple outwards from the owner's home to the community (Wood et al. 2007).

There are specific places that are more likely to attract dogs and their owners. Off-leash dog parks are the obvious example. In Australia, the distribution and maintenance of these facilities are usually the responsibility of the Local Council. Dog parks range from austere-looking fenced-in areas to whole parks dedicated to dogs, decked out with signage, waste-disposal bags and water bowls. For these places to host tension-free interactions, they need to have the same things that make any other public open space attractive. These include shading and lighting, seats for humans, access to clean and well-maintained public toilets and plenty of natural elements. Signage is particularly important in dog parks because it communicates the rules of the space and provides an opportunity for users to know what is expected—it is important that the only conflict in dog parks is the playful scrapping between the dogs, not their human companions! In addition to the provision, maintenance and regulation of off-leash dog parks, Australia's local authorities have several other responsibilities for the regulation of companion animal ownership. They manage pet registrations, take care of stray pets and enforce laws to manage inevitable pet problems (most commonly the undesirable declarations of a barking dog).

Neighbourhood streets are also spaces that host companion animals and the interactions they catalyse. The built environment correlates of dog-walking have been studied in Australia by Haley Christian, also of the University of Western Australia. Her research shows that neighbourhoods with high walkability (as described in Chapter 3—Planning for Physical Activity) also encourage people to be out and about with their dogs. Having access to a dedicated off-leash dog park is important because it gives people a place to walk to. Walking a dog in its local neighbourhood is the most popular form of public companion animal activity in Australia. However, dogs and their owners are increasingly venturing beyond the walkable catchment of their homes. Together with Corinne Mulley of the University of Sydney, Jennifer has examined the activities people do with their dogs using survey data from over 1,250 dog owners in Sydney. The study revealed that people leave their house with their dog almost half the time in a private car rather than on foot (or paw) (Kent and Mulley 2017). This practice has the potential to undermine both the social and health benefits of dog ownership by diluting opportunities for physical activity and social interaction associated with having a dog. One of the reasons people drive their dog to an outing that is beyond a walkable distance, including a trip to the vet, is because Australia has relatively strict regulations against taking pets on public transport. In Sydney, for example, a companion animal (other than an assistance dog) is not permitted to use public transport unless it is secured in a cage. This regulation ensures that a car is an essential adjunct to the practice of caring for, and appreciating, a pet.

Interaction in Neighbourhood Spaces and the Importance of Talking Points

There are many ways urban spaces can be distributed and designed to encourage incidental interactions. While we do not have the space to review them here, we recommend Jan Gehl's classic text *Life Between Buildings* (2011). First published in the early 1970s and reprinted many times, Gehl's work remains a fantastic introduction to place-making for interactions. In this section, we simplify this rich body of research to propose a very practical approach to encouraging interactions in neighbourhood spaces. Our approach is based on the provision of talking points across our towns and cities. We conceptualise talking points as both 'places to talk' and 'things to talk about'.

Talking Points as Places to Talk

Any place capable of hosting informal and unorganised social interactions in a public place is a talking point. By public we mean 'in the public realm', as opposed to publicly owned. Indeed, talking points can be a cafe or shopping mall as much as a children's playground or park bench. They can be footpaths, bus stops, bike racks or building forecourts. They can be large, such as a town square or train station, or small, such as a stairwell or common entry to a building. It seems the more talking points we have, the greater the opportunity for incidental interaction. The more often people's paths cross, the more opportunities there are to acknowledge and build respect for one another. For example, Wei Zhang and Gillian Lawson of the Queensland University of Technology surveyed activities in informal public and common places outside three high-density residential communities in Brisbane. They found that the building's common entry and the lane traversing its side were important in facilitating positive day-to-day interactions. Based on this, they recommended that the design of such spaces should be welcoming, and that the maintenance of these spaces should be prioritised throughout the building's life (Zhang and Lawson 2009).

For many, life in Australia occurs at an increasingly fast pace. The first step to an incidental interaction, therefore, might just be a slackening of pace. We need to provide a reason, and a space, for people to shift gears, even for a moment. This might be task-oriented—such as collecting the mail or waiting for a bus. It might also be rather whimsical—such as a work of public art, a body of water, a neighbourhood cat, a tree in full flower or a flock of noisy birds. Once we understand that interactions depend upon personal *de*celeration, or slowing, we realise why public spaces need to be designed to encourage lingering. The most obvious way to do this is to provide ample places for people to sit. Famous urban designer William H. Whyte was an avid supporter of the provision of seating in public places. In lamenting the lack of places to sit in American cities, he once remarked, "The human backside is a dimension architects seem to have forgotten." The quote appeared in his film *The Social Life of Small Urban Spaces* (Whyte 1980). In it, he demonstrated the way people merge and linger not in the large and exposed expanses of a public square, but in smaller parcels of space throughout the city. Aside from places to sit, there is a series of other embellishments urban planners and designers can incorporate into talking points to encourage lingering. First and foremost, they need to be places where people feel safe—a topic discussed in detail above. They also need to provide a degree of comfort. In Australia, this often means shade. On a 35-degree Celsius summer day, a bus stop that is under cover and out of the direct sun is more likely to encourage a positive incidental interaction than one that is not sheltered. To enable footpaths to host positive incidental interactions, we need to ensure they are adequately sized to accommodate the pedestrian flow. Footpaths should be accessible to those who are mobility-impaired or pushing a pram. Indeed, the fundamentals of walkability are as important for social interactions as they are for physical activity.

Talking Points as Things to Talk About

Talking points are also 'things for people to talk about'. We have already mentioned that humans share a degree of fascination with and appreciation of nature. Greenery and animals are more prone to prompt a casual remark or smile than relatively sterile blocks of concrete or steel. This is because nature is living—it is ever shifting and unpredictable. Street art—formal or informal, large or small—is also a potential talking point. Public art implores that we slow down, look up and perhaps enjoy that moment with the people who happen to be nearby. There is a multitude of ways to incorporate public art into Australia's urban environments. Given that art, in particular, should respond to the community intended to appreciate it, we do not make specific recommendations here. Instead, we once again call for a consideration of context and stress the involvement of the community in public art decision-making. We also suggest that the incorporation of artistic elements into urban elements need not be grandiose or entirely the remit of government authorities. When people dedicate time to adorning their homes with touches of their own interests and tastes, it can create points of fascination in streets that are otherwise homogeneous. This recommendation is at odds with the design guidelines often enforced by developers of new estates in Australia, which usually aspire to uniformity in building and landscape design as a way to enhance the streetscape. We propose such guides risk stifling expression, and their strict enforcement can remove opportunities for residents to shape and connect with the neighbourhood around them.

We end our discussion of talking points with acknowledgement that creation of a place to talk and things to talk about is not a remedy to draw together an isolated community. Talking points are often deeply political and contentious spaces. Rules and regulations, as well as design, can be used to both intentionally and unintentionally exclude some users. Planning for talking points, therefore, needs to go beyond simply allocating space to considering design and long-term management.

Planning for Both Sharing and Privacy

We discuss the links between urban densities and health outcomes in detail in the introduction to Part III—Domains of the Built Environment. There is a considerable body of research linking low-density development, sometimes labelled 'urban sprawl', with poor health (see, for example, Garden and Jalaludin 2009). Three of the pathways for this link is the focus on the private realm, the lack of diversity of housing types and land uses and car dependency, which can undermine social capital by reducing opportunities for social interaction. However, research on the impact of residential density on incidental interactions is mixed. Indeed, there have been several studies demonstrating that social interaction is more common in lower-density suburban areas (see, for example, the US-based study by Nguyen 2010). Overall, the research suggests that there is a threshold to be found between high and low densities and social interaction generally. People need opportunities to interact randomly, whether that be in shared driveways, building entry points or at the mailbox. But they also need to be able to retreat to private spaces from time to time.

The complex balance between density and interactions highlights the way, in Australia's densifying cities, we are increasingly required to share space. Higher-density living in an apartment, for example, replaces a private backyard with public open space. A public transport trip replaces the cocoon of the private car with a communal train, bus or tram. Australian office workers, at the mercy of employers seeking to minimise spending on office space, are increasingly asked to hot-desk, or share desk space. There are more shared pathways, where cyclists, pedestrians, dog-walkers and pram-pushers vie for space. While sharing increases the likelihood of interactions, there is some evidence to suggest that Australians struggle with the concept of sharing. The BehaviourWorks research group at Monash University in Melbourne has been applying a concept known as the Hofstede model of national cultures to some Australian practices (for example, Wynn 2018). This model, originally formulated to appraise organisational culture, contains six dimensions. It uses multiple data sources to create indices for each dimension for over 100 countries around the world. Three dimensions are of particular relevance to the concept of sharing space and facilities: power distance (respect for authority), individualism (concern for the individual over the collective good) and uncertainty avoidance (willingness to try new things). Figure 5.1 shows Australia's scores for these three dimensions relevant to Singapore and Sweden.

Australia scores low on the dimension of power distance, indicating that we generally have less respect for authority than some other nations. In other words, we are likely to consider an edict from someone in authority as a guideline or the starting point for negotiation. We score quite highly on the dimension of individualism, indicating we are less likely to prioritise the collective good over our own wellbeing. We

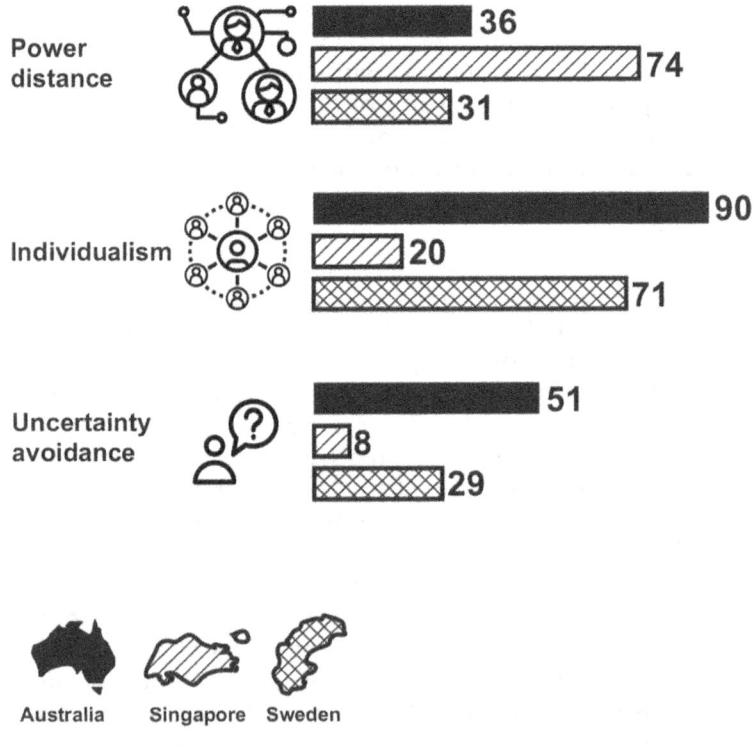

Figure 5.1 Cultural dimensions—how does Australia score?

Source: Adapted from Hofstede et al. 2010

score high on the dimension of uncertainty avoidance, suggesting we are hesitant to adopt new things. The model itself can be critiqued for being overly broad and simplistic. It fails to take into consideration the contextuality of national cultures, which are increasingly diverse and shifting faster than they ever have in the past. It only takes a few people, however, to disregard the rules (power distance) and prioritise their own needs over others (individualism) to make shared spaces less pleasant. Add to this the fact that many people are (hesitatingly) trying out new ways of living in higher density, and the need for our built environments to provide adequate and easy-to-use shared spaces becomes obvious. While planning can assist in providing adequate spaces, we can also help to educate communities about appropriate etiquette in these spaces. When people know how to behave in a space, the chance for friction amongst users is minimised and opportunities for positive, natural interaction are enhanced. This community knowledge can be developed through proper placement of signage, facilitation of educational campaigns and the provision of legible design (Gatersleben and Appleton 2007).

While sharing can encourage incidental interactions, unless sharing is balanced with the opportunity to have time out, we run the risk that interactions may become a source of tension rather than conviviality. Urban designers, in their plea to ensure that urban spaces are lively, often highlight the belief that people can make a space more liveable (Donovan 2018). In his movie, William H. Whyte, for example, remarked that "what attracts people most, it would appear, is other people" (Whyte 1980). We challenge this assumption and propose that a healthy built environment requires both opportunities for people to interact and chances for people to retreat from the public gaze when needed. As mentioned above, spaces for retreat are particularly important in higher-density developments. Planners can do this through proper building design—for example, by prioritising visual and acoustic privacy. Planners can also incorporate places for silence into everyday environments. For example, most trains servicing urban areas in Australia now have a quiet carriage, where people are discouraged from talking on mobile phones or listening to loud music. The quiet garden movement is another example of incorporating retreat into the urban fabric.

Box 5.3   The quiet garden movement

Founded in 1996, the Quiet Garden Trust is an international organisation that nurtures access to outdoor places for peace and reflection in a variety of settings. Quiet gardens vary widely in size and situation. They can be permanent, such as in a church or school setting, but can also be provisional spaces, such as the corner of a park, set aside for a particular time of day. Quiet gardens are places of hospitality—spaces for all who wish to visit. St Theodore's Church Community Spiritual Garden in Adelaide is an example in Australia. The Community Spiritual Garden uses a small pocket of land next to the church building itself. It is offered to the community as an oasis, a place of stillness and reflection, peacefulness and beauty.

Taking Interactions Online—What Place for The Built Environment?

In 1994, only 4% of Australian households had internet access (ABS 1999). By 2010, Organization for Economic Co-operation and Development (OECD) figures showed that 88.4% of Australian households were connected to the internet; this is increased from 64% in 2006. These figures are similar to comparable OECD countries, such as the United Kingdom and Canada (OECD 2018). This rise in internet connectivity has also coincided with the proliferation of mobile phone use. For a population of around 23 million people, there were almost 21 million mobile handset internet subscriptions in Australia (ABS 2015).

Increased time spent online raises the question of whether online contact can foster the types of interactions required for individual and community health. At the time of writing, the social media forums provided by Facebook, SnapChat, Twitter and Instagram were popular in Australia. WeChat is another platform used primarily by the Chinese community. In addition is the proliferation of SMS as a communication tool and the array of similar messaging apps, such as WhatsApp. The popularity of these platforms for interaction suggests that digital connections now serve as an easy substitute for face-to-face contact. This was confirmed by research from the University of Wollongong (New South Wales), which used the General Social Survey to show an aggregate decline in face-to-face contact and rise in online contact in Australia (Patulny and Seaman 2017). This is not necessarily a bad development for social interactions, which can be both initiated and strengthened by online platforms. However, it seems implausible that online interactions, self-selected and moderated by the boundaries of our own digital footprints, can provide the benefits of tangible incidental encounters with the random people around us. If we are looking down at a screen, we are certainly not looking around at the wonderful mess of community that confronts and enfolds us. Surely our ability to relate, appreciate diversity and connect to community is eroded. The question for Australia's planners, however, is whether there is any role for the built environment in moderating some of the issues that arise as a result of our appreciation of online communication.

In 2015, the United States Broadband Opportunity Council declared that the broadband internet network is taking its place, alongside water, sewer and electricity, as essential infrastructure for communities (as quoted in Middleton 2015). Assessing and approving the location and operation of major infrastructure such as water and electricity are standard urban planning concerns. Similarly, urban planning has had a substantial role to play in the provision of broadband networks across Australia. Like many other countries, Australia has recognised that a faster internet connection is now vital to people's social connections, employment prospects and ability to access services, including healthcare. In response, the Federal government has initiated the roll-out of a nationwide broadband project known as the National Broadband Network (NBN). This process started in 2009 and is expected to be completed by 2020. Research has revealed that years of political interference—and poor technology decisions—have created a prolonged state of uncertainty, both in government and the community, when it comes to this new network (Alizadeh and Farid 2017). The NBN continues to be criticised widely for being slow, expensive and obsolete. Of particular relevance to health, many have pointed to the fact that the network is not providing equitable access to broadband technology. These issues have been explored by a team at the Australian Centre for Research Excellence in the Social Determinants of Health Equity. Their research proves that Australia's areas of greatest socio-economic disadvantage overlap with regions typically receiving NBN infrastructure of poorer quality (Schram et al. 2018).

Planners in Australia assess and approve proposals for broadband infrastructure just as they do for other major infrastructure projects. The NBN relies on both underground fibre cables and satellite connections, and its construction has meant considerable disturbance to built form. Planners have overseen this process, and together with the politics and business case of the entire operation, planning decisions have had an important role in shaping the NBN. If we can use planning to influence transport networks and design new neighbourhoods, in theory, planners can also affect online networks. This raises an interesting question for healthy planning—just as we provide quiet gardens and train carriages, could we also provide spaces where access to the internet is limited to essential services? Could planners make spaces where the switched on and stressed out Australian population can genuinely find time out or genuinely find each other? In reality, Australia's planners would not dare, or be permitted, to exercise such discretion. This is a stark reminder that while we often know <u>how</u> to plan healthy built environments in Australia, the practice of planning is inevitably constrained by politics, individual preferences and the economy. These important issues are discussed further in Chapter 11—Reflections on Principles of Healthy Planning.

Conclusion

We have used this chapter on social interactions to explore the concept of incidental interactions and demonstrate their importance for healthy communities. Of course, incidental interactions are not a panacea for a disconnected community, nor can they provide immunity against serious community conflict. It is hard to imagine, however, that any urban area where it is uncommon to acknowledge, respect and care for the people around you could be a welcoming and healthy place.

What is clear from our review is that incidental interactions need space in which to occur. We have mentioned some of these spaces. However, there are many opportunities for built environments to encourage interactions, and it is impossible to cover them all here. What matters is that we continue to prioritise the provision of spaces that are welcoming and open to the public. Performing an economic or utilitarian function should not be a prerequisite for a use to claim space in our cities. By this, we mean that spaces of commerce, learning, transport, residential accommodation and service need to be complemented by spaces where use is not so well-defined—where we can linger, play, walk, sit, chat, pass through and meet. These are the spaces where "we learn—because we have to— that people of every kind, of every age, of every background deserve our respect" (Mackay 2014, p. 49).

As Australian cities grow, space comes increasingly at a premium. The business of urban development gives rise to a temptation to use every slice of available land for something deemed by the market to be 'worthwhile'. Concurrently, a growing city—and the dense urban form required to accommodate growth—demands we live in closer proximity to an increasingly diverse array of people. Spaces for interactions are, therefore, more critical than ever. These are the spaces that coax us out of our own lives and give us a place to learn to get along.

References

Aged and Community Services Australia (2015) *Social Isolation and Loneliness Among Older Australians*, Issues paper No. 1, Aged and Community Services Australia, Deakin, ACT.

Alizadeh, T. and Farid, R. (2017) Political economy of telecommunication infrastructure: An investigation of the National Broadband Network early roll-out and pork barrel politics in Australia. *Telecommunications Policy*, 41(4) pp. 242–252.

Animal Medicines Australia (2016) *Pet Ownership in Australia*, Animal Medicines Australia, Barton, ACT.

Astell-Burt, T., Feng, X., Kolt, G. S. and Jalaludin, B. (2016) Is more area-level crime associated with more sitting and less physical activity? Longitudinal evidence from 37,162 Australians. *American Journal of Epidemiology*, 184(12) pp. 913–921.

Australian Bureau of Statistics (1999) *Household Use of Information Technology, Australia, 1999*, Cat. no. 8146.0, Australian Bureau of Statistics, Canberra.

Australian Bureau of Statistics (2015) *Household Use of Information Technology, Australia, 2014–2015*, Cat. no. 8146.0, Australian Bureau of Statistics, Canberra.

Baker, D. (2012) *All the Lonely People. Loneliness in Australia, 2001–2009*, Institute Paper No. 9, The Australia Institute, Canberra, ACT.

Cacioppo, J. T., Hawkley, L. C., Norman, G. J. and Berntson, G. G. (2011) Social isolation. *Annals of the New York Academy of Sciences*, 1231(1) pp. 17–22.

Clancey, G. (2011) Crime risk assessments in New South Wales. *European Journal on Criminal Policy and Research*, 17(1) pp. 55–67.

Cozens, P. M. (2015) Crime and community safety: Challenging the design consensus, in Barton, H., Thompson, S., Burgess, S. and Grant, M. eds., *The Routledge Handbook of Planning for Health and Well-Being: Shaping a Sustainable and Healthy Future*, Routledge, London.

Cozens, P. M., Saville, G. and Hillier, D. (2005) Crime prevention through environmental design (CPTED): A review and modern bibliography. *Property Management*, 23(5) pp. 328–356.

Crocodile Dundee (1986) Film. Directed by Peter Faiman. RimStone Films.

Cutt, H., Giles-Corti, B., Knuiman, M. and Burke, V. (2007) Dog ownership, health and physical activity: A critical review of the literature. *Health and Place*, 13(1) pp. 261–272.

Donovan, J. (2018) *Designing the Compassionate City*, Routledge, New York.

Flood, M. (2005) *Mapping Loneliness in Australia*, Discussion Paper No. 76, The Australia Institute, Canberra.

Foster, S., Hooper, P., Knuiman, M., Christian, H., Bull, F. and Giles-Corti, B. (2016) Safe RESIDential environments? A longitudinal analysis of the influence of crime-related safety on walking. *International Journal of Behavioral Nutrition and Physical Activity*, 13(1) pp. 22–30.

Franklin, A. and Tranter, B. (2011) *Housing, Loneliness and Health*, AHURI Final Report No. 164, Australian Housing and Urban Research Institute Limited, Melbourne.

Garden, F. L. and Jalaludin, B. B. (2009) Impact of Urban sprawl on overweight, obesity, and physical activity in Sydney, Australia. *Journal of Urban Health-Bulletin of the New York Academy of Medicine*, 86(1) pp. 19–30.

Gatersleben, B. and Appleton, K. M. (2007) Contemplating cycling to work: Attitudes and perceptions in different stages of change. *Transportation Research Part A: Policy and Practice*, 41(4) pp. 302–312.

Gehl, J. (2011) *Life Between Buildings: Using Public Space*, Island Press, London.

Grenade, L. and Boldy, D. (2008) Social isolation and loneliness among older people: Issues and future challenges in community and residential settings. *Australian Health Review*, 32(3) pp. 468–478.

Hofstede, G., Hofstede, G. J. and Minkov, M. (2010) *Cultures and Organizations: Software of the Mind*, McGraw Hill, New York.

Kent, J. L. and Mulley, C. (2017) Riding with dogs in cars: What can it teach us about transport practices and policy? *Transportation Research Part A: Policy and Practice*, 106 pp. 278–287.

Knox, M. (2009) In retreat: Gentleman's clubs. *The Monthly*, October, www.themonthly.com.au [Accessed 11 July 2018].

Mackay, H. (2014) *The Art of Belonging: It's Not Where You Live, It's How You Live*. Pan Macmillan Australia, Sydney, NSW.

Middleton, C. (2015) Broadband is the key infrastructure for the 21st century. *The Conversation*, 30 September 2015, https://theconversation.com [Accessed 11 July 2018].

Nguyen, D. (2010) Evidence of the impacts of urban sprawl on social capital. *Environment and Planning B: Planning and Design*, 37(4) pp. 610–627.

Organization for Economic Co-operation and Development (2018) Internet access (indicator). doi:10.1787/69c2b997-en, https://www.oecd-ilibrary.org/science-and-technology/internet-access/indicator/english_69c2b997-en [Accessed 11 July 2018].

Patulny, R. and Seaman, C. (2017) 'I'll just text you': Is face-to-face social contact declining in a mediated world? *Journal of Sociology*, 53(2) pp. 285–302.

Power, E. (2016) With the rise of apartment living, what's a nation of pet owners to do? *The Conversation*, 21 May 2016, https://theconversation.com [Accessed 11 July 2018].

Saville, G. (2009) SafeGrowth: Moving forward in neighbourhood development. *Built Environment*, 35(3) pp. 386–402.

Schram, A., Friel, S., Freeman, T., Fisher, M., Baum, F. and Harris, P. (2018) Digital infrastructure as a determinant of health equity: An Australian case study of the implementation of the national broadband network. *Australian Journal of Public Administration*, 77(4) pp. 829–842.

Thompson, S. M. (2016) Animal attraction, in Architects, H. eds., *The Place Economy*, Sydney, Australia.

Ulrich, R. S. (1999) Effects of gardens on health outcomes: Theory and research, in Cooper Marcus, C. and Barnes, M. eds., *Healing Gardens: Therapeutic Benefits and Design Recommendations*. John Wiley & Sons, New York.

Umberson, D. and Montez, J. K. (2010) Social relationships and health: A flashpoint for health policy. *Journal of Health and Social Behavior*, 51(Suppl.) pp. S54–S66.

Whyte, W. H. (1980) *The Social Life of Small Urban Spaces*, Conservation Foundation, Washington, DC.

Wood, L. J., Giles-Corti, B. and Bulsara, M. (2005) The pet connection: Pets as a conduit for social capital? *Social Science and Medicine*, 61(6) pp. 1159–1173.

Wood, L. J., Giles-Corti, B., Bulsara, M. K. and Bosch, D. A. (2007) More than a furry companion: The ripple effect of companion animals on neighborhood interactions and sense of community. *Society & Animals*, 15(1) pp. 43–56.

Wynn, C. (2018) Three reasons why share-bikes don't fit Australian culture. *The Conversation*, 26 January 2018, https://theconversation.com [Accessed 11 July 2018].

Zhang, W. and Lawson, G. (2009) Meeting and greeting: Activities in public outdoor spaces outside high-density urban residential communities. *Urban Design International*, 14(4) pp. 207–214.

6   Planning for Healthy Eating

Introduction: What Is Healthy Eating and Why Is It Important?

A fresh and nutritious diet can prevent many of the common health problems facing Australians today. In fact, the major cause of morbidity in this country is now attributed to diet-related chronic disease (Australian Institute of Health and Welfare [AIHW] 2016). Health conditions associated with the way we eat include coronary heart disease, some cancers, type II diabetes and obesity. Food and the practice of eating have other implications for health, in that they present opportunities for community connection, cultural acceptance and mutual respect. Food in Australia can help define neighbourhoods, shape communities and make places.

The Australian Guide to Healthy Eating tells us that healthy foods are those that are fresh, have minimal processing and are sourced from the five main food groups: grains, vegetables, fruits, dairy and meats, fish and nuts. A healthy diet is one that involves consuming these foods each day in a balanced way (see Figure 6.1). Unhealthy diets result from disproportionate intakes of food groups, an over-reliance on processed foods and a low intake of natural, whole foods.

While these guidelines are helpful, our emphasis in this chapter is that healthy eating is all about balance. Most importantly, it is about maintaining a healthy relationship with food. By this, we mean enjoying a diversity of food experiences, meeting one's personal nutritional needs and, mostly, avoiding overindulgence in foods that lack nutritional value. In reality, many Australians struggle to find the right balance when it comes to food. The statistics on overweight and obesity are a testament to this. We know that in 2015, Australia was the fifth most obese country in the Organization for Economic Co-operation and Development (OECD) (28% of the population aged 15 and older), behind the United States (38%), Mexico (32%), New Zealand (31%) and Hungary (30%) (OECD 2017). Research examining the food Australians eat also confirms that our relationship with food is not well balanced. In 2014, 91% of people over the age of 16 did not eat sufficient quantities of vegetables,

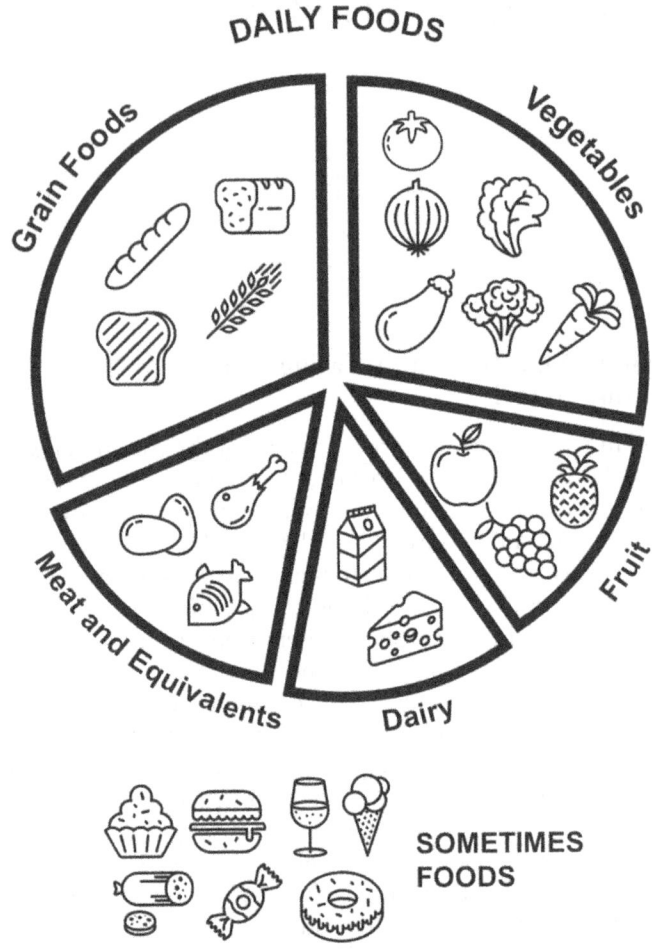

Figure 6.1 The Australian Guide to Healthy Eating

Source: Adapted from AIHW 2016

50% did not consume adequate portions of fruit and energy-dense, nutrient-poor foods made a significant contribution to the diets of children (AIHW 2016). In short, to tip the balance to a healthier food intake, Australians need to eat more fresh vegetables, fruit and grain foods, more reduced fat dairy foods, more plant-based proteins and fewer processed, nutrient-deficient foods.

How can urban planners in Australia assist with tipping this balance? Food retailing has a profound effect on dietary intake. The evidence is clear that the place where people spend most of their time, such as their neighbourhood or work environment, is a potent predictor of the food they eat (White 2007). Australia's planners shape these spaces and influence food transportation and production systems. Urban form and functioning also affect the time we have available to engage with healthy eating and, to a degree, the money we have to spend on the food we eat. The remainder of this chapter is dedicated to these issues, starting with some reflections on the structure of the Australian food system and the way Australians eat.

Healthy Eating in Australia

Food Retail Environments in Australia

As we progress through the 21st Century, the systems that provide food in Australia are shifting. Industrialisation of agriculture and increased access to global food markets have been accompanied by sociocultural changes, such as longer working hours and more time spent away from home. We now eat outside our homes regularly. These shifts have created greater demand for one-stop shopping and increased reliance on convenience and pre-prepared meals.

The most recent comprehensive data on food and nutrition in Australia was collected by the Australian Institute of Health and Welfare and published in its 2012 report, Australia's Food and Nutrition (AIHW 2012). These figures show that Australians source 63% of their food from supermarkets. A defining characteristic of the supermarket industry in Australia is that it is one of the most concentrated retail food sectors in the developed world. Two major supermarket chains, Coles and Woolworths, jointly dominate almost 80% of the market (AIHW 2012). Independent supermarkets are an alternative to the major supermarket chains, but they generally have smaller stores. Although they control only 20% of the market, these independents are an integral component of a healthy food system in Australia because they often serve regional and remote communities and have smaller networks of neighbourhood shops in urban areas. Conversely, Coles and Woolworths stores mostly occupy a large floor space and carry a huge range of products. They are usually located in major retail hubs, rather than smaller neighbourhood shopping centres, and access to them has traditionally been by private car. This has seen a decline in the number of smaller primary produce shops in neighbourhood centres. Such shops include bakeries, butchers, fruit and vegetable outlets, fishmongers and delicatessens. They are often family-owned businesses that have been unable to compete with the higher turnover, lower prices and one-stop convenience of supermarkets.

Although Australians purchase the majority of their food from a supermarket, there are plenty of places to buy ready-to-eat meals and snacks outside of major supermarket chains. Cafés, restaurants and take-away outlets now dominate shopping and other commercial centres, including within local neighbourhoods. Indeed, it sometimes seems that every imaginable use hosted by our built environment includes an opportunity to buy food. Service stations, sports matches, entertainment venues, schools, hospitals, outdoor open spaces, public transport stops, hardware stores and most public events are accompanied by food retailing, whether it be an established café, temporary stall or vending machine. And the food associated with these outlets and experiences is generally pre-prepared and highly processed, designed for easy storage and transport and on-the-spot consumption. To promote the appearance of value for money, portion sizes are often larger than what is recommended by dietary guidelines. This essentially exposes the population to endless and regular opportunities to eat large quantities of the types of foods responsible for many of the diet-related health issues dominating society today. As a result, the intense marketing and availability of foods that are unhealthy can make it very confusing for many Australians who are trying to navigate a minefield of dietary advice.

There are three interesting trends that have recently surfaced to influence the way Australians source food. The first is an emergence of an appreciation for food that is produced locally and in a manner that is more environmentally sustainable. This awareness has been accompanied by interest in farmers markets and food basket services, which deliver fresh produce to homes, as well as suburban agriculture, which is further discussed below.

The second trend has been an explosion in food delivery services more generally. In 2019, popular services are Deliveroo, UberEats and Foodora. Facilitated by online ordering technologies and the financial backing of new business models, these are services that connect homes with a variety of cafés, restaurants and take-away food outlets. Although food delivery has been available for many years in Australia, the key difference for these new services is the diversity of food offered and the fact that a company operates in between the food retailer and the consumer to facilitate the transaction. Consumers can now have gourmet meals delivered as well as traditional delivery options, such as pizza. Employees of these services are part of the 'gig economy', often paid on a per-delivery basis. They usually complete deliveries on foot or by bike or motor scooter. This practice has drawn some popular concern around employee welfare, both in terms of job security and the risks involved in walking, cycling or scooting the streets laden with food deliveries. Both of these innovations—farmers markets and online food ordering—are relatively nascent and generally operate within the geographical confines of socio-economically advantaged areas, where there is a capacity and willingness to pay for food that is both convenient and of good quality.

The final trend of interest is the emergence of discount supermarket companies that provide a challenge to the duopoly of Coles and Woolworths. Led by German retail giant Aldi, these outlets compete with the two major retailers by stocking a smaller number of goods for purchase at cheaper prices. Unlike food delivery services and farmers markets, stores are located in all socio-economic areas, usually in major shopping centres or as stand-alone outlets on the periphery of urban locales. The success of Aldi and other discount stores in unsettling Australia's food retail duopoly remains to be seen, but there are signs of shifts in consumer spending, with more shoppers electing to purchase at least some of their weekly groceries in these newer stores.

How Do Australians Eat?

Australians come to the table with different attitudes and preferences for food as well as different experiences, priorities and habits that shape when, what and where we eat. It is therefore difficult to generalise about eating practices in Australia.

We have alluded above to the fact that time stress—and the subsequent need for convenience—has changed the way Australia eats. We are increasingly eating away from home, whether it be out at cafés and restaurants, in the workplace or on the run between commitments in our cars, on public transport or while walking. Household weekly spending on meals away from home has jumped more than 55% in real terms since 1984. The majority of this growth is attributed to spending on lower-cost convenience foods (Spencer and Kneebone 2012). All three staple meals—breakfast, lunch and dinner—are now considered opportunities to eat out, accompanied by specialised menus, venues and conventions. This is a relatively new phenomenon in Australia. Prior to the 1980s, it would have been difficult to find a place away from home for breakfast; however, today, it is a common practice for many. Even when we are eating at home, we are relying more and more on pre-prepared meals or components of meals. Australians are now less likely to bake or prepare a meal from scratch, and generally we seem to have less confidence or time to spend in the kitchen. Supermarket retailers have responded to this trend with an increased supply of ready-made sauces and pastes, pre-cooked grains, pastas and meats and pre-shredded cheeses and vegetables, making cooking more a practice of assemblage than an enjoyable and creative art. A recent survey by food retailer Marion's Kitchen, for example, found that two in three Australians prefer to cook at home to save money. But it also found that despite the popularity of curries among home cooks, 82% of respondents would never make their own curry paste, and one in five could not name a single ingredient that goes into it (Ting 2013). As well as changing what we eat, being busy has led to shifts in how and when we eat. Like the United States, but perhaps different from mainland Europe, mealtimes in Australia have become increasingly blurred, with formal meals replaced by less structured snacking throughout the day. Food is less likely to be eaten at a table, with meals occurring in front of the television or other screens, at the kitchen bench, at a work desk or on the run.

These less predictable eating practices have the potential to undermine the individual's ability to adhere to dietary guidelines in various ways. Meals eaten out are more likely to be energy-dense, and meals constructed from pre-prepared ingredients are more likely to be highly processed. This has been well researched (as reviewed by Lachat et al. 2012). Serving sizes at out-of-home locations are also more likely to be larger, particularly in take-away food shops that market their goods on value for money. A study of major fast-food outlets in Australia found that, on average, a traditional fast-food meal accounted for almost 50% of the daily kilojoule guideline for healthy adults (Brindal et al. 2008). The study also found, however, that there were healthier choices available in fast-food outlets that were genuinely lower in kilojoules and more balanced. This indicates that food from the prolific take-away outlets that line our streets and dominate large shopping malls can be incorporated reasonably into a daily intake without necessarily promoting obesity. The general population, however, needs to be guided regarding these choices. We believe this education is the responsibility of the food outlets as well as health professionals and other people in positions of influence.

Another characteristic of less predictable eating practices is the deconstruction of mealtimes into more regular snacking. This also has the potential to increase food intake beyond dietary recommendations because it makes it more difficult to monitor intake across the day. Blurring the boundaries of mealtimes and locations also detracts from the ability of food to bring people together, be it family or friends, eroding what has previously been a powerful and enduring catalyst for social interaction and sharing. It is at these times that we tend to eat more slowly, enjoying a companionable experience (Dixon and Ballantyne-Brodie 2015).

Aside from being characterised by rush, convenience and commercialisation, our relationship with food in Australia has positive elements that have endured the pressures of time and the allure of the market. Being a nation of many cultures, we have come to embrace a diversity of flavours, ingredients, cooking techniques and traditions. Indeed, food has been one of the success stories of Australia's sometimes reluctant embrace of people from different countries. Food has often been used as a bridge between cultures, bringing old and new Australians together, especially helping migrants to create a sense of belonging in an otherwise unfamiliar nation (Thompson 2005).

How Can the Built Environment Provide Healthy Food Options?

Various factors influence an individual's food selection, with the planning and management of the built environment having the potential to influence them all (see Figure 6.2). For example, there are undeniable links between built environments, income and equity. Culture, education,

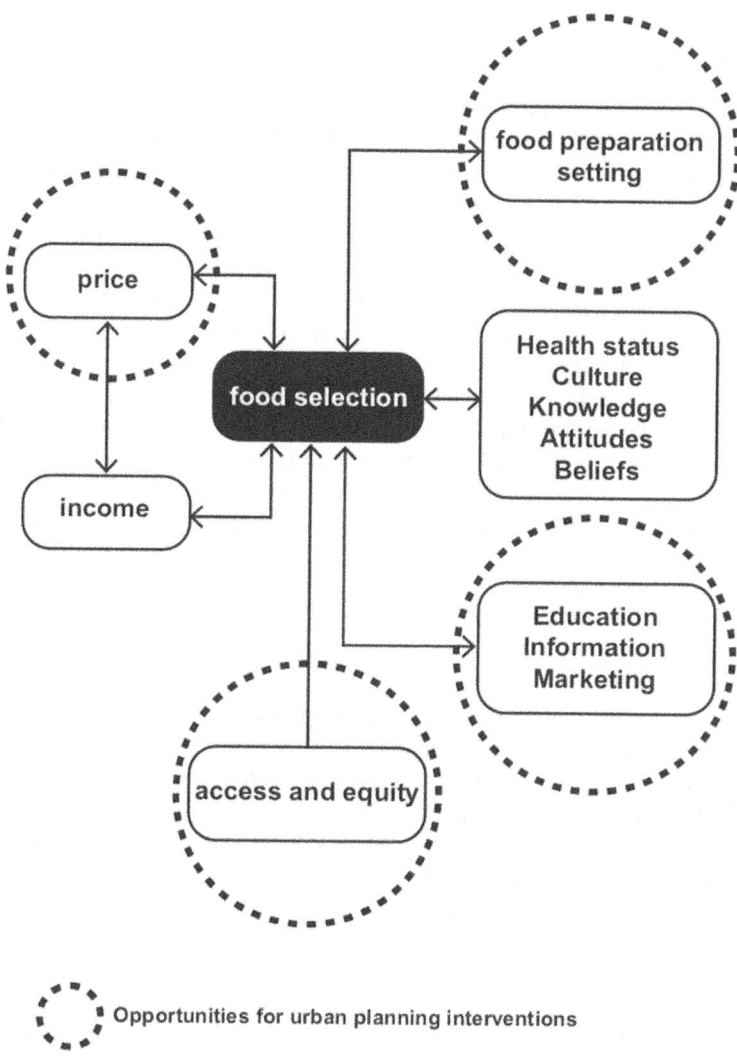

Figure 6.2 The factors that influence food choices and potential points of intervention for the built environment

Source: Adapted from AIHW 2012

attitudes and beliefs are also shaped by these environments. There are, however, some very direct ways that built environments shape food selection and these are highlighted in Figure 6.2. Firstly, our environments determine access to food, including its price and quality. Built environments also affect food preparation settings and play a part in regulating food advertising, information and marketing environments. The remainder of this chapter focuses on these more direct impacts, starting with the ways built environments shape food access and price.

Food Accessibility

Food retailers often market their products using appeals to our senses, whether it be taste, smell or sight. But in reality, research shows that the food we eat is often determined by what we can access, whether it is what we can afford or what we have time and energy to purchase and prepare.

We have established above that people who prepare food at home using fresh and less processed ingredients are more likely to incorporate variety and healthier options into their diet. Although the food available outside of the home environment varies, the research is clear that frequently eating meals and snacks bought from a fast-food shop, convenience store, café or restaurant makes it more difficult to maintain a healthy dietary intake. Land use planners in Australia struggle to address this issue. Various 'competition policies', designed to promote fair trading, prohibit planners from rejecting a business application based on the proliferation of business types already in an area. An application for a fast-food outlet, for example, cannot be refused on the basis that there are already three fast-food outlets in close proximity. This reduces the ability of urban planning to regulate the number of out-of-home food options, such as fast-food and convenience shops, in Australian neighbourhoods. It also dilutes planning's ability to regulate food sales at other venues and events, in that such regulation could be deemed to limit the appeal of the event or marketability of the venue. As well, planners cannot influence the types of foods sold in these stores, let alone temper our very human propensity to find foods that are high in saturated fat and sugar extremely palatable (Logue 2014). There are, however, some key ways that land use planners can increase the likelihood of Australians preparing healthy food at home.

Physical Access

Australia's planners can support a healthier dietary intake by ensuring that people have relatively easy, and preferably walkable, access to a supermarket. Although supermarkets are by no means devoid of less-than-healthy everyday food choices, they are the places in Australia where all the ingredients for a home-prepared and balanced meal or snack can be purchased at a relatively affordable price. Indeed, the dominance of a few large supermarket retailers has meant that most Australians now rely on the supermarket for the majority of their fresh fruit and vegetables and other staples (AIHW 2012). While there are obvious social and economic downsides to the retail duopoly that is Australia's supermarket industry, it seems that supermarkets are an important enabler of contemporary healthy eating practices. For example, as part of the RESIDE study, Georgina Trapp and colleagues from the University of Western Australia analysed the impact of behavioural, attitudinal, social and environmental influences on the food choices of 562 Western Australian residents. The findings revealed that the largest effect on healthy dietary intake was proximity to supermarkets. People in this study who lived within 800 metres of a supermarket were more likely to report a healthy dietary intake (Trapp et al. 2015). This relationship—between access to a supermarket and healthy food intake—has been the subject of intense international debate (see, for example, Ball et al. 2009). Yet the study by Trapp and her colleagues does give an Australian evidential base to the logic that we will be more likely to eat well if we can easily access a variety of affordable healthy foods. This highlights the importance of planning for mixed-use neighbourhoods so that commercial uses, such as supermarkets, can be evenly distributed throughout the city and within a walkable distance of the places where people live and work. Planning needs to support local, neighbourhood-based shopping centres rather than solely focus on the provision of larger centres designed to service more dispersed catchment areas. This is particularly important for groups less likely to have access to a private car for transporting groceries home (for example, older and younger adults [Coveney and O'Dwyer 2009]). We discuss the specific ways Australian planning can do this in Chapter 10—Commercial, Service and Employment Spaces.

On Money, Time and Energy

While supermarket access is important, our propensity to cook and eat at home is influenced by more than this. It is also a product of our willingness—and ability—to pay the various costs associated with healthy eating. While these costs are monetary, they also involve the investment of time required to source and prepare healthy food. The time and monetary cost of healthy eating will be personal. Willingness and ability to pay are shaped by socio-economic, demographic, cultural and structural factors. The way our cities are planned and managed, however, can also influence these things.

In terms of monetary cost, international research consistently finds that in most countries, it is more cost-effective to source food from a supermarket and prepare it at home than rely on convenience food options (Wilsher et al. 2016). The Federal Department of Agriculture, Forestry and Fisheries examined the food chains in Australia and found that this generally applies (Spencer and Kneebone 2012). There are, however, variations in the cost of foods in Australian supermarkets. Healthy food is generally less available and more expensive in some areas, particularly in rural and remote Australia (AIHW 2012). Indeed, the socio-economic gradient to poor health is sometimes positioned as related primarily to healthy food being expensive and difficult to purchase in socio-economically deprived and geographically isolated places. The debate linking socio-economic status and accessibility to healthy food has subsequently informed the development of the concept of food deserts—conceptualised as places where cheap and varied food is inaccessible by any transport mode other than the private car (Macintyre 2007). Although the actual existence of food deserts continues to be debated, Australian research has attempted to quantify and qualify the relationship between the location of food outlets, socio-economic status and poor health. This research generally finds that residents of lower socio-economic status neighbourhoods in Australia have the poorest access to supermarkets. For example, a study in Melbourne (Ball et al. 2009) found that people living in more advantaged neighbourhoods had a greater number of supermarkets and fruit and vegetable stores within two kilometres of their home.

Like the residents of many countries around the world, Australians are spending more and more time working and commuting. Our sprawling urban landscapes mean that precious snippets of time between conflicting commitments are often dedicated to rushing across increasingly congested cities. This quality of day-to-day life makes the convenience of access to food within our immediate surroundings an even more important determinant of food choices and patterns of consumption. Indeed, lack of time to purchase and prepare healthy food is often cited as a barrier to healthy eating (Coveney and O'Dwyer 2009) and one that seems to have been passed down to younger generations (Crawford et al. 2010). This is a common theme throughout our book. For example, time availability impacts the propensity to be physically active and socially connected. This sense of time scarcity has similar implications for healthy eating. Urban planning has a role to play in slowing down our speeded-up society by bringing uses such as schools, homes and employment opportunities closer together, thereby helping to ensure that our spare time is not spent battling congestion. In relation to facilitating time to eat healthy food, the planner's best recourse is to ensure that we have multiple opportunities to access key ingredients. As mentioned above, this is about giving people access to healthy food within their local neighbourhoods.

It may seem obvious, but cooking and eating at home are possible only if we have access to decent kitchen facilities. This has recently come to the fore in some of Australia's capital cities, where apartment design guidelines have enabled flats to be built with minimal provision for kitchen space (George 2016). Deprivation of facilities for cooking and storing food is also a key risk factor associated with crowded dwellings, an issue addressed in Chapter 7—Residential Spaces.

Fostering a Positive Relationship With Eating and Food

Cooking at home requires certain skills and confidence, and these are attributes that can be developed through education and exposure to a culture that celebrates fresh and healthy food. Growing fresh food at home, participating in community gardening and frequenting farmers markets are examples of practices where the appreciation of fresh produce can be fostered. Many of these practices rely on suburban agriculture, and urban planning has a role to play in ensuring the success of these uses across Australia. More succinctly, suburban agriculture includes the use of pockets of space within our built-up areas as well as larger tracts of land in our cities to grow food. It includes community gardens, rooftop vegetable patches and the use of verge space between the footpath and road for food production. It is an increasingly popular concept in Australia. A recent survey of 1,390 people indicated that more than half of Australian households are involved in growing their own fresh food (Wise 2014). The emergence of a renewed cultural appreciation of locally and sustainably produced food has added further momentum to the embrace of farming activities across our cities and suburbs (see Box 6.1). Suburban agriculture provides many health benefits, including opportunities for physical activity and social connections, and this has been well researched in Australia (see, for example, the work of Cumbers et al. 2018). Importantly, farmers markets and community gardens also provide healthy food options. They increase the availability of fresh vegetables and fruit and inspire an appreciation of food that has been locally produced. Farmers markets in particular can also increase competition at nearby food stores, lowering the price of fresh produce in these outlets.

An appreciation of healthy eating starts in childhood, and one of the most disconcerting impacts of the way we consume food today is the toll it takes on children. One in four Australian children is currently considered overweight or obese (AIHW 2017). It is therefore worthwhile giving some consideration to the way food is sold and marketed in and around the places where children spend their time, particularly schools. 'School food environments' are conceived as the food provided within the school as well as outlets serving foods within the vicinity. While urban planners in Australia have little sway over the interior food environment of schools, planning processes can, through land use zoning and regulation, influence the types of uses near educational establishments, including the density of fast-food outlets. Some localities in the United States have bravely passed laws to prohibit the co-location of fast-food restaurants and school uses (see Reeve et al. 2015 for a review of local policies in the United States). Australia, however, has not yet embraced this as an option. Local Councils attempting to regulate the placement of fast-food outlets face various legal and political constraints, including charges of over-regulation and anti-competition, as well as a lack of evidence and resources to engage in court-based settlements Reeve et al. 2015. There is scope for these challenges to be met with empirical evidence, a harnessing of community concern for childhood obesity and better policy design.

As urban planners working at the intersection of planning and health, we are mindful of the need for food to be positioned in society as a positive and life-giving force, rather than an emotionally charged entity to be demonised and feared. In examining the links between urban planning and healthy eating, researchers rarely interrogate the relationship between what we eat and how we are feeling. The ways our cities are planned and managed are undeniable shapers of our emotional state, and emotional eating is often a precursor to overeating. By providing ample, safe and well-designed green, open and community spaces, as well as ensuring our cities are equitable and responsive to context, Australia's urban planners can defuse the stress of modern life. Well-planned cities can reduce the need for unhelpful stress outlets, including binge eating, restrictive dieting, over-exercising and drinking to excess. Our message is that built environments need to promote choice and balance in eating practices, where health, rather than simply convenience or a quick fix, determines the food we eat.

Box 6.1   Urban agriculture in Melbourne

Urban agriculture thrives in Australia's second largest city, Melbourne. The city is alive with community gardens and food cooperatives as well as farmers markets, food waste initiatives and food banks.

This embrace of urban agriculture in Melbourne is the result of a mix of environmental and cultural conditions that have changed over time. The city has favourable biophysical conditions for growing food. It is located on fertile soils, in a temperate zone, with a reliable water supply. Until the post-war era, most households produced some kind of fruit and vegetables or kept livestock, particularly chickens. The 1950s heralded the rise of multinational supermarkets, and 'low-maintenance' gardens became more popular. A flood of immigrants from Southern Europe in the 1960s and '70s brought a renewed enthusiasm for vegetable gardening and the keeping of livestock in the suburbs. The emergence of the environmental movement in the 1970s further encouraged domestic food production in Melbourne as a means of generating greater self-reliance. From this time onwards, Melbourne's dispersed and extensive geographical layout has fostered a landscape of community gardens and urban farms, including the Collingwood Children's Farm (established in 1979) and the Community Environment Park (known as CERES, founded in 1982). These farms operate alongside several community-growing programs, including Cultivating Community (founded in 1998), the Stephanie Alexander Kitchen Garden Project (founded in 2001) and the Asylum Seeker Resource Centre (founded in 2001).

Source: Edwards 2011

Planning the Built Environment and Food Production

The need to preserve farming on the peri-urban lands around large cities is increasingly recognised in Australia (Mason and Knowd 2010). While Australia is a vast and relatively unpopulated country, much of its land is unsuitable for large-scale agricultural production. Areas that have access to sufficient water, arable soils and protection from climate extremes are generally around the periphery of the nation. Yet these are also the areas where most Australians live.

In an effort to absorb unrelenting population growth, Australia's arable lands have consistently been rezoned from agricultural to urban uses. This is often at the expense of food production, resulting in the steady decline of locally produced fresh fruit and vegetables (Mason and Knowd 2010). Unfortunately, this is a trend that is set to continue as Australia's cities grow. In Melbourne, for example, it is estimated that the peri-urban region has the capacity to meet approximately 41% of the city's current total food needs. To accommodate forecast growth, however, it is predicted this figure will fall by 18% by 2050 (Carey et al. 2016).

A sensible approach, and one that has ironically been at planners' fingertips for a while, is to use land use zoning and regulation to protect peri-urban agricultural lands. This strategy reduces the need to transport produce long distances and therefore has co-benefits for health and the biophysical environment. These co-benefits are increasingly relevant in the context of climate change, as we discussed in Chapter 3—Planning for the Health of the Planet. Using the urban fringe for agriculture, however, poses particular difficulties for Australia's planners. It requires an approach to development that seeks to use existing areas in ways that are more efficient, usually implying increased urban densities. The planning mechanisms and impacts of increased densities in Australian cities are discussed throughout this book, particularly in the introduction to Part III—Domains of the Built Environment.

As discussed above, urban planners also have a role to play in supporting an emergent cultural (re)embrace of suburban agriculture. Many of these ways of growing food require the oversight of urban planners, who influence the allocation of land for different uses across the city through the function of land use zoning. This important planning function simply means that all land across an area is allocated a specific zone, such as residential, commercial or recreational. It originated in the 19th Century out of the need—and ability—to separate unhealthy, polluting uses from the places where people lived. It was originally a direct response to the Industrial Revolution, which brought with it both an upscaling of noisy, smelly and dirty uses to be avoided and the emergence of new ways to travel relatively long distances away from these uses. As a result, our urban areas today are made up of a mosaic of zones. Within each zone, certain uses are permitted and others are prohibited. If a piece of land is zoned as commercial, for example, that land can be used for a shop but not for a house or a hospital. While this might seem logical to us today, to those living in housing scattered amongst the factories and tanneries of Manchester in the 1800s, it would have been quite radical. It is the zoning function of planning that regulates suburban agriculture, meaning we cannot just grow and sell food anywhere we like in Australia's urban areas. Instead, we have regulations that attempt to ensure food-related activities occur only in areas where such use is compatible with the surrounding uses. Incompatibility might relate to safety. For example, in some places it is prohibited to locate a community garden on a main traffic-generating road because of concerns about contamination of produce as well as the safety of gardeners. It could also be related to amenity. For example, in some areas local produce cannot be sold on the roadside because of worries about additional traffic and parking generation. These are two fairly obvious examples, but problems arise when definitions of what is safe and amenable differ within the community. Does a verge planted out with an overenthusiastic pumpkin vine detract from or enhance the visual appeal of the streetscape? Should a locality embrace a roadside produce stall even if it means that traffic is slowed and parking is less available? In Australia, these are generally issues that are the responsibility of Local government. Planners resolve them by developing new policies and regulations to respond to changing demands or by assessing applications for food-growing and distribution uses on a case-by-case basis. Many Australian cities are currently growing and densifying quite rapidly, and growing one's own produce is enjoying a renaissance. Accordingly, it is not surprising that some local authorities are dealing with conflicts as they juggle differing community aspirations within traditional planning regulatory regimes.

This struggle is potentially the result of local authorities failing to acknowledge that they have a key role in supporting sustainable and healthy food systems. There are immense benefits—biophysical, economic and social—to be gained from the prioritisation of urban agriculture. Yet there is evidence that food is not a Local government priority in Australia. Strategic planner Jan Fallding has undertaken a comprehensive review of the way health was framed as a Local government issue across New South Wales (Fallding 2016). Her content analysis of community strategic plans was commissioned by Active Living New South Wales. She found that only 10% of strategies mentioned anything about food systems as a priority. Surprisingly, most of these came from rural Local Councils, who saw food security and the opportunities presented by local food production as urgent concerns. There is obviously room for our metropolitan Local Councils to catch up and capitalise on the increased cultural interest in farming our suburbs.

Conclusion

This chapter has shown that we are more likely to eat healthy food if it dominates our retail choices, is relatively inexpensive and is easy to source, store and prepare. This is increasingly relevant in our speeded-up societies, where time is often a scarce resource.

We have examined the way Australians are now eating away from their homes more and eating in a way that is increasingly unstructured. This has an impact upon dietary intake in several ways, not least because meals eaten out are generally more kilojoule-dense and less nutritious than food prepared at home. Also, most Australians do not eat the recommended daily serves of vegetables and fruit. There are many ways Australian urban planning can help people engage more with cooking and eating at home and ensure that their food intake better reflects national dietary guidelines. Firstly, we can guarantee people have physical access to places to purchase good quality and affordable produce. Usually, in Australia, this will be at a supermarket, which should be within a walkable distance of where people live and work. It is therefore important for planners to safeguard the smaller-scale shopping centres that once thrived in our local neighbourhoods. Finally, we discussed the way urban planning supports local food production. This includes protecting periurban agricultural lands from development and encouraging people to grow their own food in community gardens, on verges and in their own yards or on their balconies.

This is the final chapter in Part Two—Domains of Wellbeing. This Part has covered the way good urban planning can address some of the key risk factors for poor health facing Australia. We started with the undeniable foundation of a healthy population—a healthy planet. We then covered several activities key to wellbeing that are supported by this planet.

Physical activity, social interaction and healthy eating are all practices that planners can, and do, influence in Australia, and we hope our discussion here has clearly articulated these pathways. In the next Part—Domains of the Built Environment—we address the built outcomes required to support health and wellbeing in Australia.

References

Australian Institute of Health and Welfare (2012) *Australia's Food and Nutrition 2012: In Brief*, Cat. No. PHE 164, Australian Institute of Health and Welfare, Canberra, ACT.

Australian Institute of Health and Welfare (2016) *Australia's Health 2016*, Australian Institute of Health and Welfare, Canberra.

Australian Institute of Health and Welfare (2017) *A Picture of Overweight and Obesity in Australia*, 2017, Cat. no. PHE 216, Australian Institute of Health and Welfare, Canberra, ACT.

Ball, K., Timperio, A. and Crawford, D. (2009) Neighbourhood socioeconomic inequalities in food access and affordability. *Health & Place*, 15(2) pp. 578–585.

Brindal, E., Mohr, P., Wilson, C. and Wittert, G. (2008) Obesity and the effects of choice at a fast food restaurant. *Obesity Research & Clinical Practice*, 2(2) pp. 111–117.

Carey, R., Larsen, K., Sheridan, J. and Candy, S. (2016) *Melbourne's Food Future: Planning a Resilient City Foodbowl*, Victorian Eco-Innovation Lab, The University of Melbourne, Melbourne.

Coveney, J. and O'Dwyer, L. A. (2009) Effects of mobility and location on food access. *Health & Place*, 15(1) pp. 45–55.

Crawford, D., Cleland, V., Timperio, A., Salmon, J., Andrianopoulos, N., Roberts, R., Giles-Corti, B., Baur, L. and Ball, K. (2010) The longitudinal influence of home and neighbourhood environments on children's body mass index and physical activity over 5 years: The CLAN study. *International Journal of Obesity*, 34 pp. 1177–1187.

Cumbers, A., Shaw, D., Crossan, J. and McMaster, R. (2018) The work of community gardens: Reclaiming place for community in the City. *Work, Employment and Society*, 32(1) pp. 133–149.

Dixon, J. and Ballantyne-Brodie, E. (2015) The role of planning and design in advancing a bio-nutrition-sensitive food system, in Barton, H., Thompson, S., Burgess, S. and Grant, M. eds., *The Routledge Handbook of Planning for Health and Well-Being: Shaping a Sustainable and Healthy Future*, Routledge, London.

Edwards, F. (2011) Small, slow and shared: Emerging social innovations in urban Australian foodscapes. *Australian Humanities Review*, 51 pp. 115–134.

Fallding, J. (2016) *A Baseline of Healthy Eating and Active Living Within NSW Local Government Community Strategic Plans and Selected Delivery Programs*, New South Wales Premier's Council for Active Living, Sydney, NSW.

George, B. (2016) Yes, but what's it like to live there? Part 3: Better apartment design standards? Not yet. *Planning News*, 42(9) pp. 15–16.

Lachat, C., Nago, E., Verstraeten, R., Roberfroid, D., Van Camp, J. and Kolsteren, P. (2012) Eating out of home and its association with dietary intake: A systematic review of the evidence. *Obesity Reviews*, 13(4) pp. 329–346.

Logue, A. W. (2014) *The Psychology of Eating and Drinking*, Routledge, London.

Macintyre, S. (2007) Deprivation amplification revisited: Or, is it always true that poorer places have poorer access to resources for healthy diets and physical activity? *International Journal of Behavioral Nutrition and Physical Activity*, 4(32).

Mason, D. and Knowd, I. (2010) The emergence of urban agriculture: Sydney, Australia. *International Journal of Agricultural Sustainability*, 8(1–2) pp. 62–71.

OECD (2017) *Obesity Update 2017*, OECD Publishing, Paris.

Reeve, B., Ashe, M., Farias, R. and Gostin, L. (2015) State and municipal innovations in obesity policy: Why localities remain a necessary laboratory for innovation. *American Journal of Public Health*, 105(3) pp. 442–450.

Spencer, S. and Kneebone, M. (2012) *FOODmap: An Analysis of the Australian Food Supply Chain*, Department of Agriculture, Fisheries and Forestry, Canberra.

Thompson, S. M. (2005) Digestible difference: Food, ethnicity and spatial claims in the city, in Guild, E. and van Selm, J. eds., *International Migration and Security: Opportunities and Challenges*, Routledge, Milton Park.

Ting, I. (2013) How Australia eats: The ultimate pie chart. *Good Food*, 5 November 2013, www.goodfood.com.au [Accessed 26 May 2018].

Trapp, G. S., Hickling, S., Christian, H. E., Bull, F., Timperio, A. F., Boruff, B., Shrestha, D. and Giles-Corti, B. (2015) Individual, social, and environmental correlates of healthy and unhealthy eating. *Health Education & Behavior*, 42(6) pp. 759–768.

White, M. (2007) Food access and obesity. *Obesity Reviews*, 8 (Suppl. 1) pp. 99–107.

Wilsher, S. H., Harrison, F., Yamoah, F., Fearne, A. and Jones, A. (2016) The relationship between unhealthy food sales, socio-economic deprivation and childhood weight status: Results of a cross-sectional study in England. *International Journal of Behavioral Nutrition and Physical Activity*, 13 p. 21.

Wise, P. (2014) *Grow Your Own: The Potential Value and Impacts of Residential and Community Food Gardening*, Policy Brief No. 59, The Australia Institute, Canberra, ACT.

Part III

Domains of the Built Environment

Introduction

Part III of *Planning Australia's Healthy Built Environments* transitions from healthy behaviours to healthy built form. We identify four 'Domains of the Built Environment'. In a healthy planning paradigm, these are the backdrops for good health. They are the structures and systems that allow us to minimise the harm of risk factors such as physical inactivity, social isolation and environmental devastation.

We start with residential spaces, recognising the significance of not only the structure but also the concept of home for human wellbeing. We then outline the importance of public and open space as a vital component of the city that, if managed properly, can promote many elements of human health. Chapter 9 turns to networks, with a focus on the health impacts of transport, including the complex relationship between health and private car use in Australia. The final chapter has its focus on some of the more diverse—and sometimes under-considered—spaces that make up urban Australia. We concentrate on three that we regard as integral to a healthy built environment: employment spaces, healthcare spaces and school spaces. For each chapter, we explore some of the ways these Domains of the Built Environment impact upon health, then examine the Australian response to their provision.

Prior to progressing to specific Domains of the Built Environment, we take time to examine the critical concept of density. Density is both a planning process and an outcome, and it permeates all aspects of the relationship between built environments and health. Recognising this, we believe that it is unwise to connect the concept of density to any one particular built environment domain. It is often conceptualised as relevant to the residential domain, yet its impact and constituent parts relate just as much to open space, places of employment and transport networks. This examination, therefore, is often referenced throughout our text, reflecting the complex yet critical role of density in planning Australia's healthy built environments.

A Note on Density

Defining Density

In urban planning, density is the quantity of a particular unit (or units) per an area of land. Units can be houses, jobs, people, amenities, infrastructure or an array of other elements of the built environment. An area of land might be an individual lot, a neighbourhood, suburb or city, or it could be a more empirical measure, such as metres squared or hectares. For example, in Australia, we may say that the residential density of a typical suburb is 15.5 dwellings per hectare.

Discourse on density is common in healthy planning practice and research. This is because a healthy built environment is both dependent upon and vulnerable to the impacts of density. Planners and health practitioners are particularly interested in residential density because many of the health benefits and risks associated with density are actualised in the realm of the home. Neighbourhoods are often described as being low-, medium- or high-density (see Figure Part III.1). We stress, however, that for density to have health-promoting effects, it needs to be considered as more than just residential density.

What Is It About Density?

Many of the elements of a healthy built environment—such as neighbourhood-based shops and services, public and active transport infrastructure, green open spaces that are well maintained and even community events—require a critical mass of people to make them possible. This is firstly because these elements require economic investment, which can be justified only if there are people who will benefit from and use them (a local supermarket or a new bus route are good examples). Secondly, these things need people to bring them to life. Parks, footpaths and community gardens feel safer, are more likely to be cared for and are more convivial if they have a reliable and regular user base. Thirdly, in a very complex way, density is linked to transport. There is undeniable empirical evidence that lower-density urban areas—such as those that dominate Australian cities—will struggle to transition away from private car dependency. This complexity is woven through concepts such as distance, destinations, land use diversity and the design of infrastructure. These are commonly known as some of the 'Ds' that feature in alternative transport discourse. We cover them in detail in both Chapter 4—Planning for Physical Activity—and Chapter 9—Transport, Access and Health.

Having established that density is a key variable in making healthy built environments work, we must also caution that too much density can have detrimental health impacts. Concepts such as overcrowding epitomise this. The place we call home, however, does not necessarily

LOW DENSITY

0-25 dwellings per hectare
usually single residential housing

MEDIUM DENSITY

25-60 dwellings per hectare
town-houses or three to five storey
apartment blocks

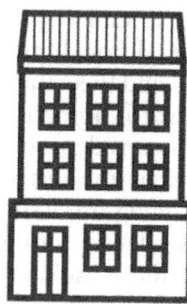

HIGH DENSITY

+60 dwellings per hectare
usually apartment buildings over
three storeys

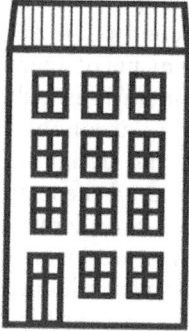

Figure Part III.1 Residential density definitions suggested for Australian urban
areas

Source: Adapted from Udell et al. 2014

need to be overcrowded with people for us to feel unsettled by things
such as diminished privacy, the need to compete for everything from a
seat on a train to a child's turn at the swings and the inability to escape
the rush and busyness that are increasingly characteristic of modern life
in Australian urban areas. These are subtle experiences that are only
just beginning to be unearthed by the research. Studies to date highlight
the isolating impact of 'too much' density on vulnerable populations,
such as the elderly (Giles-Corti et al. 2012). Others point to the dis-
advantages associated with raising a family in an apartment building

that is not designed to accommodate active children (Whitzman and Mizrachi 2009).

How Much Density Is Enough?

In attempting to balance the benefits with the costs of density, planners and health professionals are often compelled to ask, *how much* density is enough? Indeed, the idea of 'proper city densities' (Jacobs 1961, p. 221) has been the subject of debate in planning theory and practice for quite some time, although its relationship with health is a more recent topic of discussion and theorisation. At the risk of frustrating policy makers' insatiable thirst for numerical quantification, we suggest that better solutions arise from consideration of three key aspects of density.

The first is the distribution of residential densities relative to other uses, including infrastructure, services, open space and other amenities. A medium-density double storey apartment block that is of poor construction and is isolated from essential services, including public transport, will be far less supportive of a healthy lifestyle than a ten-storey apartment building that is built for longevity and is within walking distance of shops, transport, schools and green space.

The second is the design of the building. We discuss some of the key design elements of apartment buildings in Chapter 7—Residential Spaces. Key considerations include designing for acoustic and visual privacy and designing to accommodate a diversity of household types. Quality construction and design are also important for higher-density built form's ability to stand the test of time.

The final consideration is the existing context of the area. To accommodate population increases and encourage a transition towards more sustainable ways of living, Australian planners and communities generally recognise the need for increased density. Often this is pursued through policies of urban consolidation—a growth management approach that aims to increase density in existing built environments. Unfortunately, there are many examples in Australia where planners have failed to manage this densification process properly. Too often residential amenity has been compromised, the public domain neglected and the character of existing neighbourhoods ignored. Reduced privacy, increased noise levels, worsening road traffic and overcrowded on-street parking and green space within neighbourhoods are commonly cited issues (Byrne et al. 2010). Planners often fail to recognise that density is a relative concept, and its impact on an existing community will depend on the acquired experiences, skills and understandings of the community undergoing consolidation. In Australian cities transitioning towards increased density, many community groups, urban activists and some scholars have criticised urban consolidation. Although, as mentioned above, poor planning is often at the heart of these criticisms, they are also founded on the fact that densification requires change, which can challenge deep-seated feelings of belonging as your familiar local neighbourhood is transformed. Those living in and near density may never have experienced the benefits—or drawbacks—of being part of a larger, more animated community. This must be acknowledged and considered for healthy higher density to become a reality in Australian cities.

References

Byrne, J., Sipe, N. and Searle, G. (2010) Green around the gills? The challenge of density for urban greenspace planning in SEQ. *Australian Planner*, 47(3) pp. 162–177.

Giles-Corti, B., Ryan, K. and Foster, S. (2012) *Increasing Density in Australia: Maximising the Health Benefits and Minimising the Harm*, National Heart Foundation of Australia, Melbourne.

Jacobs, J. (1961) *The Death and Life of Great American Cities–The Failure of Town Planning*, Penguin Books, Middlesex.

Udell, T., Daley, M., Johnson, B. and Tolley, R. (2014) *Does Density Matter? The Role of Density in Creating Walkable Neighbourhoods*, National Heart Foundation of Australia, Melbourne.

Whitzman, C. and Mizrachi, D. (2009) *Vertical Living Kids: Creating Supportive High-Rise Environments for Children in Melbourne*, University of Melbourne, Australia, Melbourne.

7 Residential Spaces

Introduction: What Do We Mean by Residential Spaces?

Australia's built environments are primarily residential. Our cities and towns are characterised by the buildings and streets that constitute 'home' for Australia's people. This chapter is about the way our homes—including the neighbourhoods around them—influence health in Australia.

How Do Residential Spaces Influence Health?

Australian cultural geographer Robyn Dowling introduces her co-authored text on home with the following statement:

> 'Home' is a significant geographical and social concept. It is not only a three-dimensional structure, a shelter, but it is also a matrix of social relations and has wide symbolic and ideological meanings. Home can be feelings of belonging or of alienation; feelings of home can be stretched across the world, connected to a nation or attached to a house. The spaces and imaginaries of home are central to the construction of people's identities.
>
> Blunt and Dowling 2006 (cover copy)

This statement demonstrates that although the impact of home on health is undeniable, it is also infinitely complex and multilayered. It starts with the very air we breathe. The place where we live conditions this air. Our homes determine the degrees to which our bodies are exposed to variations in temperature, whether we feel warm on days and nights when it is colder outside and cool throughout the long, hot Australian summer. The dwelling also shapes our exposure to contaminants, both from the materials comprising the building, its fittings and fixtures and from the environment around us. On another level, simply having a place to call home, where one feels a sense of belonging and refuge, is important for health. A secure, safe and well-maintained home grounds us and gives us a place from which to plan, prepare and prime ourselves for more obvious healthy behaviours, such as preparing healthy food or being physically active. The location of home also has an impact on health, as it determines access to services, employment and health-promoting infrastructure such as green open spaces and networks for cycling and walking. Finally, in Australia, housing is a major financial investment. It is a marker of status that can be passed from one generation to the next. The security of home ownership is therefore particularly embedded in our culture, and this has complex and lasting impacts on our health.

This multilayered view of the impact of home on health is internationally acknowledged in academic and policy literature. To examine these layers in an Australian context, we view the health impacts of residential spaces as related to the following elements:

- Housing design
- Housing adequacy
- The place around home
- Tenure
- Housing affordability

Housing Design

Housing design refers to the interior and exterior structure of the home. Design affects the way a home feels—for example, enabling adequate ventilation and privacy from neighbours. It also influences the way a home looks, which in turn shapes how we feel and act within that place. Importantly, housing design also impacts the amount of space, and sometimes also the time, we have available to engage in health-promoting or demoting practices, including physical activity, social interaction and healthy eating.

The design of residential spaces regulates indoor air temperature and quality. The links between these factors and health are well researched in the Australian context. Indoor temperatures and air quality are associated with many physical health outcomes, particularly respiratory conditions, with children and the elderly especially vulnerable. People who cannot afford to heat or cool their homes mechanically are also more at risk. Although not strictly speaking Australian, research by Philippa Howden-Chapman and colleagues in New Zealand illustrates this well (Howden-Chapman et al. 2007). Their study used a longitudinal randomised controlled study design to evaluate the health impact of installing insulation in housing. They found that adults in insulated homes were half as likely to report respiratory complaints (such as wheezing and coughing) and winter colds and flu as those without insulation. While the sample was not representative of the general New Zealand population, the results do demonstrate the way interventions to regulate indoor air quality, such as proper insulation, have a significant effect on physical health.

In Australia, protection from heat is of paramount importance, particularly given the rising temperatures associated with global warming and the urban heat island effect. This is discussed in Chapter 3—Planning for the Health of the Planet—where we point out the health implications of heatwaves, which are an increasingly common occurrence during our prolonged summers. Poor quality housing and social isolation are both implicated in epidemiological studies on the links between heatwaves and health (Coates et al. 2014). Low-income households are particularly vulnerable because they have fewer options for responding to heatwave events. Poor quality housing generally heats up quickly, retains heat and is less likely to be fitted with air-conditioning. Restrictions on what public and private tenants can do to their home to make it more comfortable when the weather heats up are also problematic. As well, lower-income households are more likely to be located away from the protective sea-breezes of coastal locations (Yardley et al. 2011). Finally, social isolation increases vulnerability to adverse health outcomes from hot weather because of the inability to reach out and seek help, or travel to places to escape the heat (such as shopping centres or cinemas).

A major strategy for reducing the risk of illness or death from heatwaves has been the widespread adoption of air-conditioning in Australian homes. Fifty years ago, only 10% of Australian homes had air-conditioning, compared with 75% today (Australian Bureau of Statistics [ABS] 2014). Of course, this growth can be partly attributed to advances in technology and affordability. However, the changing climate and poor dwelling construction practices, together with cultural expectations of comfort, are also implicated. Studies of heatwave health outcomes have shown that air-conditioning in homes is a protective factor mitigating negative health outcomes. Retrospective research indicates that the presence of air-conditioning in the home reduces heat-related illness by approximately 80% (Nicholls et al. 2017). This is compared with an electric fan, which reduces illness by only 30%. Indeed, air-conditioning is increasingly promoted by Australia's health authorities as the most effective way to prevent heat-related illness. This has significant equity implications. Indeed, highlighting the vulnerability of low-income households in increasingly hot weather, multiple Australian studies demonstrate the way low-income households restrict their use of air-conditioning. For example, a study of welfare-dependent, aged people found that they even limited their use of low-power electric fans (Waitt and Farbotko 2011). A similar study conducted in Western Australia revealed that 60% of low-income survey respondents restricted their use of heating or cooling despite bodily discomfort (Cornwell et al. 2016). These studies point to the concern in Australia regarding the high cost of energy supply to households as well as sufficient supply during periods of peak demand, particularly at the peak of summer. Climate change is increasing the duration and intensity of Australia's extreme heat events. This lays bare the vulnerability of our energy supply and demands reduced reliance on fossil fuel–generated electricity. The logical response is to pursue construction of houses that are more resilient to severe weather through the use of energy-efficient design and siting (Nicholls et al. 2017). The ways Australia is planning for more climate-responsive homes will be discussed further in the second part of this chapter.

Designing to Enable Personal Control

Visually, the internal design of housing impacts upon aspects of mental health, which in turn affects our ability to engage in other healthy practices. Interior home design can promote a sense of calmness and tranquillity or invigoration and engagement. Colours, shapes and sounds can stimulate in different ways, producing various health outcomes. A key to ensuring that the interior design of a home is healthy is that its inhabitants have some control over various stimuli. This includes exposure to sources of noise as well as light and the extent and location of personal items and embellishments. As with so many factors discussed in this book—and relevant to the built environment's impact on health—the extent and type of exposure may not be as important as the individual's ability to shape and control that exposure.

An Adequate Home

Healthy homes provide a balance of opportunities for household members to interact (such as in open-plan kitchens and living areas) as well as retreat. In addition to space for cooking, eating and sleeping, a healthy home will provide space for other key functions, such as washing, studying, playing and relaxing. A lack of adequate space, often referred to as overcrowding, is related to poor mental health outcomes, including anxiety and depression. Overcrowding also influences health because of its impact on living practices, such as being able to store and prepare healthy food, ensure a healthy standard of cleanliness and obtain a restful night's sleep.

In Australia today, we know surprisingly little about the extent of chronically overcrowded housing in our urban areas. Formal analyses of housing conditions define overcrowding as whether the dwelling provides an adequate number of bedrooms for different household configurations (see the Canadian National Occupancy Standard in Figure 7.1 as an example). A 'severely overcrowded' dwelling is defined as one in which four or more additional bedrooms are needed to accommodate the residents of that dwelling sufficiently. For example, a dwelling requiring

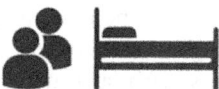

no more than two people should share a bedroom.

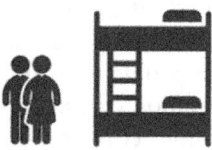

children of different sexes under five years of age may reasonably share a room.

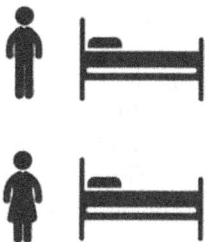

children of different sexes should not share a bedroom when aged five or older.

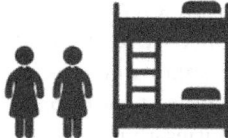

children under 18 and of the same sex may reasonably share a bedroom.

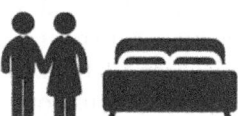

parents, couples and household members aged 18 or older should have a separate bedroom.

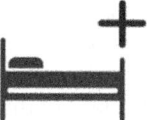

households that need at least one extra bedroom are considered to be experiencing some degree of overcrowding.

Figure 7.1 Defining overcrowding using the Canadian National Occupancy Standard

Source: Adapted from Mallett et al. 2011

four extra bedrooms would be a two-bedroom flat shared by 12 people! Australian researchers and housing practitioners include those living in 'severely crowded' dwellings in counts of the homeless population. In 2016, 44% of our homeless population nationwide was deemed 'homeless' because they were living in severely crowded dwellings (ABS 2018). This is a problem of mounting concern amongst the general population in our major cities. Increasing housing costs, particularly high rents, are driving people to share actual bedrooms with strangers in order to live in proximity to the jobs, education and services they need to access within the city. The increasing popularity of short-term rentals advertised through online platforms such as Airbnb is exacerbating this issue. Data from the University of Sydney's Urban Housing Lab, for example, calculates that in 2016, about 6,000 properties in Sydney were removed from the rental market and offered to higher-paying tourists (Gurran and Phibbs 2017).

While formal analyses define overcrowding as whether the dwelling provides an adequate number of bedrooms for different household configurations, we know that regardless of access to a bedroom, a dwelling can feel small and inadequate for our needs. This is particularly so if indoor and outdoor spaces do not provide sufficient privacy or space for the activities that make up day-to-day life. For example, we may have space to sleep but lack access to appropriate cooking and washing facilities or spaces to study and congregate. Definitions of what is crowded will also differ according to our previous experiences, culture and age. It is therefore possible that a home can feel crowded to the extent that it influences our health without necessarily fitting the official definitions of 'overcrowded' used by the Australian government.

Regardless of definitions, an increase in crowding and related lack of privacy and ability to withdraw from the pressures of day-to-day life are of growing concern to those experiencing increases in residential density. Our introduction to Australia's cities (see Chapter 1—Australia and Australia's Planning) revealed a general consensus for the need to increase density to accommodate growing populations in a more sustainable, and hopefully healthier, way. We explored the way sprawling, low-density development is associated with several unhealthy aspects of city living, including private car dependency. In addition to ensuring that higher-density development is well served by public transport and other infrastructure, such as schools and places of employment, the design of higher-density development will be key to its ability to promote the health of those who will one day call these spaces home. There are many ways to ensure that higher-density developments do promote health, ranging from well-written Strata Title laws that encourage peaceful and cooperative close living, to the siting of bedrooms and other principal living areas away from main roads and other noise-generating uses. Some of these design guidelines will be discussed in the second half of this chapter.

The Residential Place

Our homes do not exist in isolation from the wider urban area in which they are located. This includes the physical neighbourhood around the dwelling and extends to the way homes are linked to the broader opportunities provided by the city, including access to employment, transport infrastructure and other services.

The Design and Function of the Immediate Neighbourhood

The immediate neighbourhood around people's homes has abundant capacity to support health. Streets provide the background for simple physical activities such as walking and children's play. These spaces are for the meeting and greeting of neighbours and passers-by, and they are a canvas for practical and fun expressions of personalisation and sharing. The external spaces immediately surrounding the buildings we call home are our interface with the social world. As such, they affect the way we view and treat that world. Their design can set the stage for an ongoing relationship with society and an environment founded on respect and mutual understanding. Street design, safety and neighbourhood trimmings are three key elements.

Neighbourhood street design: The actual layout and use of streets in residential areas influence our behaviour, including whether we walk, talk or play there. Australian research shows that street networks supporting a high level of permeability and connectivity are more likely to be those where people walk, both for recreation and transport, and where people are out and about in the neighbourhood (Christian et al. 2017). This does not necessarily mean the more traditional grid street patterns. Indeed, one qualitative study conducted in Melbourne, Victoria, found that the cul-de-sac, often discouraged in healthy planning design guides, encouraged children's neighbourhood-based play (Veitch et al. 2006). What seems to matter is that streets are designed to maximise safety and provide a sense of legibility. With regard to pedestrian safety in residential areas, traffic should be slowed, with the pedestrian given priority. In relation to legibility, the streets for homes should be easy to navigate and set out in a way that is predictable. This encourages exploration of the residential neighbourhood on foot.

Safety: We know that people will not interact within or feel part of a community they perceive to be unsafe. Our health suffers as a result. Yet there are many personal, social and built factors that contribute to whether one feels safe in one's neighbourhood. In Chapter 5—Planning for Social Interaction—we introduced the concept of Crime Prevention Through Environmental Design, or CPTED. In summary, this is an umbrella term for physical interventions to the local environment and built form aimed at improving safety from crime. Many of the components of CPTED are operationalised at the neighbourhood scale to ensure the spaces around homes are safe. For example, the maintenance of infrastructure (including footpaths and landscaping), and provision of adequate lighting, can prevent creation of areas of concealment. As well, siting residential buildings to face the street enables casual surveillance from front rooms, verandahs and balconies, which enhances safety and a feeling of security in the neighbourhood.

Neighbourhood trimmings: The smaller details of the design and operation of residential places have immense importance in promoting a sense of attachment to where we live. This is critical for health both directly to support good mental health and indirectly to ensure that people feel confident and comfortable being physically active and involved in their neighbourhoods. Residential places need to be well maintained and have footpaths of adequate width for walking, street trees for shade and lighting at night. In addition to these basic treatments, there is a large body of research suggesting that people are more likely to be out and about in residential places if they perceive them to be aesthetically pleasing. The subjectivity of appeal makes this a challenging concept in healthy built environment research. For some, the attraction of a neighbourhood may have more to do with, for example, the types of buildings it hosts or the views it enables. For others, garden verges and a soundscape enlivened by the noise of birds and other wildlife will be important. While aesthetically pleasing places are significant for health, beauty, in particular, is 'in the eye of the beholder', and any evaluation of the aesthetic quality of a place is destined to be subjective. This is particularly relevant in Australian towns and cities, which are often comprised of a mosaic of cultural heterogeneity. The key for urban planning is to incorporate diversity into place-making decisions, a challenge discussed further in Chapter 11—Reflections on Principles of Healthy Planning.

Location Relative to Other Uses and Activities—Siting

Most literature on healthy built environments promotes the need for residential buildings to be intermixed with other uses, such as shops, schools, services and community facilities. This recommendation is based on the idea that the closer these destinations are to people's homes, the more likely they are to access them on foot (Gunn et al. 2017). One way to ensure this proximity is to mix things up. Placing other destinations amongst residential uses also gives people a reason to be out and about in their neighbourhood, which encourages social interaction. Ways to plan for a diversity of uses, as well as desirable destinations, will be covered in detail in Chapter 10—Transport, Access and Health. In summary, because most Australian urban areas grew at a time when car use dominated, planners (and the voting public) saw little need to reduce distances between uses or to mix those uses up. In fact, until quite recently, planning in Australia has been quite rigid in enforcing strict zoning controls and has discouraged intermingling of uses relative to other developed nations. As a result, most of our suburbs demonstrate relatively little mixing, epitomised by the fact that many suburban households do not live within a walkable distance of a small shopping centre. Planning for health in Australia must continue to discourage the homogeneous swathes of residentially zoned land that have traditionally characterised our cities.

Tenure

Australians are historically attached to the notion of home ownership. Approximately 65% of us either own our home outright or are paying off a mortgage (ABS) 2017). This long-standing trend has only recently been challenged by increasing house prices, rendering home ownership an unaffordable prospect for many, particularly younger people. Indeed, the rate of home ownership among 18- to 39-year-olds across Australia declined from 36% in 2002 to 25% in 2014. In the same age group, the decline in home ownership has been largest for families with dependent children, falling from 56% to 39% (Wilkins 2017). Nevertheless, home ownership remains a cultural aspiration and social norm. Interestingly, research in Melbourne suggests that those who 'fit' this norm are actually more likely to report better self-rated health (Badland et al. 2017).

Outside the two dominant types of tenure—owning and renting—only 1.6% of Australians live in social housing. This is a very low proportion relative to many European countries. In Australia, government authorities manage the majority of social housing stock, commonly known as public housing. A large and diverse group of not-for-profit organisations also own and manage a small proportion of social housing, known as community housing. Over time, the focus of social housing in Australia has moved away from supplying affordable properties to low-income working families towards providing accommodation to households with special needs or in challenging circumstances. While social housing in Australia does offer an important safety net for households unable to secure housing in the private market, experts in this space generally agree that both the social housing stock and the system that allocates it to those in need are inadequate (Randolph et al. 2018).

Security of tenure, whether it be through ownership or a stable rental arrangement, is an important but indirect means by which housing—and planning—influences health. This aspect of healthy housing has been well researched in the Australian context by a series of projects funded by the Australian Housing and Urban Research Institute (AHURI). These Australian-based studies generally agree that owner-occupation is the 'healthiest' tenure type (for example, Goodman et al. 2013 and Hulse et al. 2014). There are several pathways linking home ownership to health. International research has demonstrated that home ownership is associated with higher psychosocial wellbeing (Kearns et al. 2000) and lower risk ratios for mortality across a range of common causes (Breeze et al. 1999). Many privately owned houses will be in better physical condition, and this surely explains some of the relationship. Homeowners, however, are also documented as experiencing an increased sense of security, which is associated with better health (Hiscock et al. 2001). Residential security is measured by encounters with the traumatic experience of a forced move. This is more likely to occur for tenants in private rentals. However, the contours of insecurity for private renters are incredibly complex, extending beyond experiences of forced relocation (see Morris et al. 2017 for a review of this complexity in an Australian context). This is further discussed below.

Affordability

When housing is deemed to be unaffordable relative to household income, we say that a household is experiencing 'housing stress'. Judith Yates, an economist and Honorary Associate Professor at the University of Sydney, has spent many years researching housing affordability in Australia. She defined a rule of thumb to identify housing stress known as the '30/40' rule. This rule defines a household as experiencing housing stress if housing costs are greater than 30% of household income for those in the bottom 40% of the income distribution (Yates et al. 2007). According to this definition, various analyses suggest that approximately 7% of Australian households are officially experiencing housing stress. We know, however, that many more households are struggling to pay their rent or mortgage even though they may not officially be experiencing housing stress.

The unaffordability of housing in Australia is regularly the subject of media reports and social commentary. Indeed, it has become somewhat of a cultural obsession, particularly in major cities, where housing is increasingly expensive. And while health might not be the focus of our obsession, health statistics show that Australians have reason to be concerned about the cost of housing. Although the links between housing affordability and health are complex, there is no doubt that experiences of housing stress are related to poor health outcomes. Many of these health impacts stem from a lack of stability and sense of control over the living environment, with the health outcomes the same as those related to insecurity of tenure outlined above. Spending a large proportion of income on housing can also inhibit an individual's ability to maintain healthy practices because the money is simply not available. This might include seeking medical attention, buying and storing healthy food and even prioritising the purchase of basic attire and equipment that can make physical activity such as walking comfortable, safe and enjoyable.

Having considered different ways in which residential spaces influence health, we now move on to discuss how we can positively plan for health-supportive residential streets, neighbourhoods and towns. We start with a focus on healthy housing.

Planning for Healthy Residential Spaces in Australia

Planning for Healthy Housing

There are internationally prescribed guidelines around what constitutes a house that is safe and healthy. In Australia, these guidelines are mandated through a set of minimum building standards known as the National Construction Code (NCC). The NCC mandates technical requirements for not only safety and health but also amenity and sustainability in the design and construction of buildings throughout Australia. The ability for the NCC to shape health outcomes associated with residential dwellings cannot be overestimated; however, this is often overlooked in the healthy planning literature. The NCC establishes performance criteria for factors such as insulation, ventilation, room sizes, ceiling heights and access to sunlight as well as the general standard of construction quality that must be met, including ensuring a home is safe. This in turn determines the quality and longevity of the building, which affects not only the residents of the building itself but also the look and feel of the surrounding neighbourhood. A street hosting a series of well-designed buildings constructed with care should remain habitable for many years to come. In contrast, a series of poorly constructed dwellings can start to show signs of dilapidation and age relatively soon after initial occupation. This decay influences the way residents feel both in and about the place where they live, which inevitably affects their sense of mental and physical wellbeing.

While the NCC is internationally recognised as adequate, its application to producing quality, healthy housing outcomes has been questioned on several fronts. Firstly, while builders of faulty dwellings (those not compliant with the code) face legal and financial ramifications, many faults do not appear for several years post construction. Yet in most States, builders of new homes need guarantee their work for a period of just six years for major defects and 24 months for those that are minor. Secondly, following a global trend in Local government reforms, Australian States have now shifted to allow private businesses to monitor and certify compliance with the NCC. All new buildings are examined for compliance with the NCC and other policies both during and post construction. In short, until the early 1990s, most homes were certified by the Local government authority. Although practices do differ from State to State, Australia's home builders now have the option to employ a private certifier. There is evidence suggesting that not all certifiers in Australia perform their roles with the experience and health of the end user in mind (Drane 2015). This is worrying, as certifying authorities have considerable power to ensure that the residential building approved for construction is what is actually built. While very little empirical data exists on the gaps between buildings approved and those constructed, anecdotal evidence suggests that this could be a potential loophole through which the promise of healthy residential spaces could easily slip. This clearly requires further research in the Australian context. A final potential area of weakness in the application of the NCC is the significance of the construction sector for the Australian economy. As a result, constraining cost growth and improving productivity to support economic growth have been a primary concern in the development and modification of the NCC. It is easy to see how these economic concerns could easily override the need to provide a premium standard of built form, which we would argue is essential for good health.

Most State and Territory jurisdictions augment the NCC with other design guidelines and controls. These additional controls also have a huge capacity to increase the health-promoting qualities of residential buildings. For example, in Victoria, new apartment buildings must comply with both the NCC and the Better Apartments Design Standards. These standards were implemented in early 2017 in response to community and professional concerns about apartment buildings having bedrooms without windows, kitchens too small for proper meal preparation and insufficient provision of private and communal open space. The new standards prescribe many of the components of healthy buildings, including minimum requirements for cross-ventilation, storage and access to daylight from habitable rooms. Still, a space remains in Australia for a national healthy residential building standard. Such regulations are in place elsewhere. For example, the United Kingdom Green Building Council published the Health and Wellbeing in Homes Report in 2016 (UK Green Building Council 2016). A potential mechanism for this in Australia would be to tap into existing tools used to mandate development of more energy and water-efficient houses. Several advances have been made in this space. Federally, the Green Building Council maintains a Green Star rating system to assess the sustainable design, construction and operation of buildings, fitouts and communities (see Chapter 3—Planning for the Health of the Planet—for further details). State governments also maintain policies for building sustainability, which, in some cases, have the added bonus of being legislatively mandated. For example, in New South Wales, all applications for new dwellings or substantial amendments to existing houses need to comply with a policy known as BASIX. A critical concern here, however, will be addressing situations where a home's sustainability performance potentially undermines its ability to be a comfortable and healthy place to live. Earlier in this chapter, we mentioned the link between air-conditioning and reduced risk of morbidity and mortality from heatwaves and sustained periods of above average temperatures. The use of air-conditioning in homes is discouraged in sustainability guidelines because it is so energy-intensive. This is an example of a conflict that will need to be resolved if sustainability indices for housing construction and renovation are modified to incorporate health considerations. A role certainly exists for educating the occupiers of sustainable buildings on ways to optimise new technologies and unfamiliar designs for healthier outcomes.

A final, yet important, limitation to the use of building standards to deliver healthy residential spaces is the inability to apply such standards retrospectively. The exception is in extreme circumstances where a dwelling poses a fire or other risk. Accordingly, it is the responsibility of the owner to maintain a home that has healthy design features. A lack of awareness, economic resources or practical knowledge leaves many people vulnerable to living in unhealthy housing, particularly those in rental accommodation, who have little control over repairs. This vulnerability is augmented in Australia because of a history of poor quality housing construction. For example, many of Australia's established suburbs are dominated by detached dwellings constructed during the long boom experienced in cities after World War II (see Chapter 1—Australia and Australia's Planning). With money in short supply, over a third of Australians opted to build their homes themselves during this period. In the absence of regulatory safeguards, this meant that many homes were built by inexperienced and untrained individuals. As an example of the decline in quality, before World War II, most Australian homes were of timber or double brick construction. The high cost of double brick eventually led to the development of homes made of brick veneer. This is an internal timber structure covered with a single external layer of brick. This construction method has endured, with many new Australian homes still constructed using brick veneer. While modern construction systems ensure that homes use insulation products in the floors, walls and ceiling, not all homes have been retrofitted in this way. Poorly constructed examples remain relatively common throughout established suburbs, making many of our homes hot in summer and cold in winter. The planning system has little power over this because there is no regulatory mechanism to retrofit existing housing to ensure that it provides a higher standard of comfort and health.

Planning for Security of Tenure and Permanency

Many of the health-promoting aspects of built environments either depend on or are strengthened by a sense of permanency in the residential environment. Familiarity, predictability and a connection to the place where one lives can enable the etching out of time and emotional space required to lead a happy and healthy life. Security of tenure and a sense of permanency in the place we call home are critical determinants of health.

For most Australians unable, or unwilling, to invest in the purchase of a home, private rental accommodation is the main option for securing a place to live. There are several reasons why renting in Australia is practised and perceived as an insecure housing model. Firstly, and perhaps related to an historical and culturally embedded prioritisation of home ownership, the regulation of the rental market in Australia is less robust than in some countries where renting is more common. Australia's renters face substantial housing insecurity, with 50% on a fixed-term one-year lease and 20% on a month-to-month 'rolling' lease. Secondly, in most States, the legislation governing rental arrangements currently allows for 'no-grounds eviction'—that is, a tenant can be evicted at the end of a fixed-term lease or during an ongoing lease without reason. This situation is juxtaposed with some European countries, such as Germany, where rental laws hold that eviction can only be enforced if there has been violation of a lease agreement (Martin et al. 2018). Thirdly, Australian tenants are also limited in what they can do to personalise their rented home. Landlords can refuse any request from a tenant to make cosmetic changes to a property (such as hanging a picture), keep a companion animal or even alter a property to allow an older person or person with a disability to live there (Power 2017).

In addition to ensuring security of tenure, there are other ways planning in Australia can achieve permanency and a sense of continuity in a neighbourhood. The first is adaptability. Housing needs to be responsive to future societal needs as well as evolving economic and environmental conditions. This is particularly the case for Australia's ageing society, where 'ageing in place' is considered of primary importance in ensuring a healthy and high quality of life into old age. Planning has a role to play in ensuring adaptability, not least by taking an adaptive and flexible approach to zoning and design guidelines. Most local development controls now specify that a certain percentage of new dwellings need to be adaptable to accommodate people with limited mobility and other disabilities. The NCC also contains standards for adaptable housing. Secondly, planning in Australia can encourage quality building practices. Housing for health must be well-designed and constructed using quality materials. There are residential spaces that will be, by their nature, not settled by a permanent community. A good example is the student housing increasingly dominating the neighbourhoods around Australia's universities. These buildings can still be planned to promote a sense of permanency and care by ensuring quality construction that stands the test of time.

Planning for Affordability

While entering the housing market is an embedded and, until recently, assumed Australian social aspiration, monumental increases in housing prices, particularly in major cities, have ensured that this aspiration is unlikely to become a reality for many Australians. As house prices have risen, so too have rents, and there are many more renting households in stress than home-buying households. As discussed above, perhaps of greater concern is that as many as 100,000 Australians are currently homeless (ABS 2018). How, therefore, can we plan for affordability and equity of access to secure housing in Australia?

If affordability is at the heart of security of tenure, the supply of housing is at the heart of affordability. Our cities are growing, and without new dwellings, the law of economics deems that increased demand for housing will lead to increased house prices. Until the early 21st Century, the supply of new dwellings in Australia generally kept pace with demand. A combination of shrinking household sizes and increasing populations, however, has meant that there is a growing gap between supply and demand, resulting in increases in house prices.

Although by no means primarily responsible, planners are implicated in the decrease in affordability in Australia. Through the power to rezone land as residential and to increase the density of residential areas, urban planning has a role to play in ensuring adequate supply of land for residential development. This also means that urban planning determines the housing mix that can be provided on a parcel of land by regulating density, height and siting. A greater housing mix—that is, the provision of apartments, townhouses as well as detached dwellings—increases affordability through the delivery of a variety of housing options. This includes options at lower price points than would be the case if, for example, our suburbs continued to be dominated by single block houses. Another lever for planners in influencing housing price is through the provision of infrastructure. When infrastructure, such as public transport and schools, is provided for an area, the cost of housing in that area increases. By ensuring that everyone has access to the kinds of infrastructures in demand, planners can contribute to the 'levelling out' of housing markets.

It is important to note, however, that urban planning can only contribute to the easing of housing affordability (Gurran and Phibbs 2013). Planners are just one component of a very complex and powerful housing 'machine' that is driven by a series of other institutions and stakeholders, including developers, construction companies, fiscal policies and politics. Other factors shaping housing supply and affordability in Australia include a tradition of favourable taxation regimes for investors, a lag in dwelling and apartment construction despite planning approvals, community opposition to increased density and, in some cases, a lack of infrastructure to make development a viable proposition.

The planning system also plays a role in the supply of social housing for those in most need. As outlined above, this is known as public or community housing, and Australia performs poorly in its provision and management (Pawson et al. 2016). Planning approaches to the provision of affordable housing include the maintenance and protection of existing affordable housing but in some cases extend to government-produced and owned affordable housing. In contemporary Australia, most new public housing is provided by private developers, who deem a small percentage of the dwellings that are constructed to be affordable and entrust management of these dwellings to a community housing provider. Expanding waiting lists for this type of community housing and increasing homelessness suggest that this is not an effective system. More needs to be done to ensure that a social housing safety net exists to provide shelter for people when they need it.

Planning for Better Designed Residential Spaces

There are many great resources developed to articulate the more specific components of healthy residential spaces in Australia. Some of these are listed in Appendix Two—Four of Four. The key challenge that remains in Australia is how to interpret these guidelines into plans and built form so that healthy neighbourhoods can be developed on the ground. We discuss these challenges in Chapter 11—Reflections on Principles of Healthy Planning. To conclude this chapter, we present two case studies of planning where health promotion through the built environment was an articulated goal. We use these case studies to present stories of both successes and lessons learnt.

Case 1: Oran Park, New South Wales

Oran Park is a 300-hectare site located 60 kilometres southwest of Sydney's central business district. When complete, the estate will house over 21,000 people. Most will live in free-standing houses; however, there is also provision for some apartments and terrace houses. Future plans also provide for 50,000 square metres of retail and 150,000 square metres of commercial floor space. In addition, the proposed final estate will contain three schools, new administration headquarters for the Local government authority, Camden Council, a retirement village, a library, an aquatic centre and an integrated healthcare facility.

As part of the South West Priority Growth Area in Sydney, Oran Park was subject to a special precinct planning process, which included the release of a Structure Plan, an Indicative Layout Plan and finally a Development Control Plan containing the more minor controls for the development (known as a DCP). At the beginning of the planning process, there were limited references to healthy planning provisions. The general idea of 'walkable neighbourhoods' was mentioned in the structure plan for the broader region (known as the South West Growth Centre Structure Plan), but no specific health objectives were included. Planning at the DCP level provided the most specific measurable guidelines for development in relation to health. The vision for the site reflects this: "the Oran Park Precinct will establish itself as a high-quality urban environment founded on the principles of community pride, well-being, healthy living and educational excellence" (Department of Planning and Environment 2016, p. 15). The DCP contains both general objectives and specific controls for the site, some of which are based on the Heart Foundation's *Healthy by Design* guidelines (Heart Foundation 2004). General objectives related to the delivery of healthy residential neighbourhoods include the provision that the majority of residential lots be located within 400 metres' walking distance of an existing or proposed bus stop. Specific controls include the condition that all dwellings be located no further than 400 metres from a public park and that minimum requirements be provided for off-street shared cycle and pedestrian pathways. The controls also mandate that trees are required on every street.

It is too early to evaluate whether the health provisions written into the plans for Oran Park have benefitted residents' health. In 2018, Jennifer undertook some preliminary work on the connectivity of the site to the wider metropolis of Sydney and the impact of transport provision on residents' ability to use active transport. This work found that while the internal design of the precinct is highly walkable, once residents leave Oran Park, they are forced to do so in a private car. While most residents live within walkable distance of a public transport stop, the frequency of services and connectivity to the wider network are inadequate to stimulate regular use (Kent 2018). This work highlights the need for healthy built environments to look beyond the design of the immediate neighbourhood. In many cases, the neighbourhood's location relative to commonly accessed destinations—in particular, places of employment—will be as important in encouraging healthy practices.

Case 2: The Liveable Neighbourhood Code, Western Australia

The Liveable Neighbourhood Code is a development control policy designed to improve the health and wellbeing of residents of new developments in Western Australia (Western Australian Planning Commission 2015). It specifically promotes more compact, interconnected neighbourhoods that reduce car dependency and encourage walking, cycling and public transport use. The code is designed to be applied to three scales of residential development and must be considered in regional and district structure plans, local structure plans and individual subdivisions. It has eight elements: community design, movement network, lot layout, public parkland, urban water management, utilities, activity centres and employment and schools. Each element is comprised of two components: key objectives (description of aims) and requirements (qualitative and quantitative responses to meeting the objectives). Requirements are phrased as either "matters that *must* be satisfied" or "matters that *should* be considered". The key difference is that the former are mandated, whereas the latter are merely encouraged. Most matters in the Code relating to health fall into the second 'should' category. For example, provisions relating to walkability, such as ensuring that the majority of residents live within 400 metres of a public transport stop, are a "matter that *should* be considered". Grid-like street networks, important for walkability, are also in this category.

The application of the code has been researched extensively by a team led by Billie Giles-Corti, now at RMIT University in Melbourne. Known as the RESIDEntial Environments Project (often shortened to RESIDE), the landmark study used a longitudinal design to investigate the application and outcomes of healthy built environment principles. Professor Giles-Corti has gone on to lead Australian empirical research in this space. Her work is highly cited and has placed Australia on the international landscape in data-driven analysis of health and the built environment.

There are multiple publications reporting the findings of the RESIDE study. We recommend the article on walkability published by Christiansen et al. (2016) as a good entry point. The team's findings relating to actualisation of the policy through the on-the-ground planning of residential developments are particularly interesting. They found that only 47% of 42 policy requirements had been implemented. They also identified several barriers to the implementation of the policy, including a lack of clarity about requirements and the need for more rigorous enforcement through the planning approval process. The status of Liveable Neighbourhoods as an operational policy rather than a State Planning Policy (which provides the highest level of planning control in the State of Western Australia) is also considered a limitation.

Case Study Summary

These two cases demonstrate that the barriers to creating healthy home environments in Australia exist at different scales. In Oran Park, the precinct reflects some important elements of healthy built environments, and these elements were included because of their specific articulation in the planning controls applicable to the development. The controls did not, however, adequately consider the way the area is positioned and linked relative to other uses, and as such it is our sense that Oran Park will be a car-dependent community. In RESIDE, connections to the wider region were considered because the Liveable Neighbourhood requires application at regional, local and site scales. It seems, however, that barriers were faced in implementation, with many of the health-promoting components of the Code failing to be applied.

These are just two case studies of residential developments seeking to incorporate healthy planning principles in Australia. There are many others, published both in the scholarly literature and by key organisations in the healthy planning space in Australia, including the extremely useful Healthy Active by Design site maintained by the Heart Foundation (2018). We stress that case studies such as these are important records for those seeking to promote healthier residential spaces.

Conclusion

We opened this chapter on residential spaces by emphasising that the concept of home has wide symbolic and ideological meaning. The place we call home shapes our health in many and varied ways. The physical design of the building provides shelter and conditions the air we breathe and the temperatures we experience. Having a safe and secure home, with a sense of permanency and control, is also a central component of residential spaces that influences personal health and wellbeing. Finally, the location of the home relative to other activities, such as work, shapes the amount of time and energy we can dedicate to healthy practices, including being out and about in our neighbourhoods.

Home ownership has traditionally been an important social and economic aspiration in Australia. Other tenure types, such as renting, continue to be culturally and institutionally positioned as somehow inferior. This is reflected in regulations that favour the security of the landlord over the rights of the tenant. It is against this background of cultural aspirations for home ownership that house prices in many of Australia's largest cities have increased exponentially. At its worst, this housing affordability crisis has resulted in an increase in homelessness and overcrowding. Although not as influential on health directly, the lack of affordable housing in our major cities is provoking an overwhelming sense amongst many Australians that housing is precarious. This perception inevitably influences wellbeing by diminishing the individual's sense of security as well as eroding attachments to place and community. High housing costs also mean that many individuals and families must forgo expenditure on practices of care, including physical activity and nutritious food.

By promoting affordable housing options and providing safe, attractive and tension-free residential neighbourhoods, urban planning in Australia can attenuate some of the effects of our relatively unbridled housing market. We believe this is one of the most significant roles for planning in health promotion in Australia today. It is one that needs to look beyond micro-design elements, such as footpath widths and grid-like streets, and towards the role of planning in wider structures of provision, including economics and politics.

References

Australian Bureau of Statistics (2014) *Environmental Issues: Energy Use and Conservation*, Cat. no. 4602.0.55.001, Australian Bureau of Statistics, Canberra, www.abs.gov.au [Accessed 28 July 2018].

Australian Bureau of Statistics (2017) *2016 Census QuickStats*, Australian Bureau of Statistics, Canberra, http://quickstats.censusdata.abs.gov.au/census_services/getproduct/census/2016/quickstat/036 [Accessed 28 July 2018].

Australian Bureau of Statistics (2018) *Census of Population and Housing: Estimating Homelessness, 2016*, Cat. no. 2049.0, Australian Bureau of Statistics, Canberra, www.abs.gov.au [Accessed 28 July 2018].

Badland, H., Foster, S., Bentley, R., Higgs, C., Roberts, R., Pettit, C. and Giles-Corti, B. (2017) Examining associations between area-level spatial measures of housing with selected health and wellbeing behaviours and outcomes in an urban context. *Health and Place*, 43 pp. 17–24.

Blunt, A. and Dowling, R. (2006) *Home*. Routledge, London.

Breeze, E., Sloggett, A. and Fletcher, A. (1999) Socioeconomic and demographic predictors of mortality and institutional residence among middle aged and older people: Results from the longitudinal study. *Journal of Epidemiology and Community Health*, 53(12) pp. 765–774.

Christian, H., Knuiman, M., Divitini, M., Foster, S., Hooper, P., Boruff, B., Bull, F. and Giles-Corti, B. (2017) A longitudinal analysis of the influence of the neighborhood environment on recreational walking within the neighborhood: Results from RESIDE. *Environmental Health Perspectives*, 125(7) pp. 077009.

Christiansen, L. B., Cerin, E., Badland, H., Kerr, J., Davey, R., Troelsen, J., van Dyck, D., Mitáš, J., Schofield, G., Sugiyama, T., Salvo, D., Sarmiento, O. L., Reis, R., Adams, M., Frank, L. and Sallis, J. F. (2016) International comparisons of the associations between objective measures of the built environment and transport-related walking and cycling: IPEN adult study. *Journal of Transport and Health*, 3(4) pp. 467–478.

Coates, L., Haynes, K., O'Brien, J., McAneney, J. and de Oliveira, F. D. (2014) Exploring 167 years of vulnerability: An examination of extreme heat events in Australia 1844–2010. *Environmental Science and Policy*, 42 pp. 33–44.

Cornwell, A., Hejazi Amin, M., Houghton, T., Jefferson, T., Newman, P. and Rowley, S. (2016) *Energy Poverty in Western Australia: A Comparative Analysis of Drivers and Effects*. BCEC Research Report no. 2/16, Bankwest Curtin Economics Centre, Curtin University, Bentley, WA.

Department of Planning and Environment (2016) *Oran Park Precinct: Development Control Plan*, NSW Department of Planning and Environment, Sydney, NSW.

Drane, J. (2015) Building defects how can they be avoided? A builder's perspective. *Strata and Community Title in Australia for the 21st Century Conference*, 2–4 September 2015, Gold Coast, Queensland.

Goodman, R., Nelson, A., Dalton, T., Cigdem, M., Gabriel, M. and Jacobs, K. (2013) *The Experience of Marginal Rental Housing in Australia*, AHURI Final Report No. 210, Australian Housing and Urban Research Institute Limited, Melbourne.

Gunn, L. D., King, T. L., Mavoa, S., Lamb, K. E., Giles-Corti, B. and Kavanagh, A. (2017) Identifying destination distances that support walking trips in local neighborhoods. *Journal of Transport and Health*, 5 pp. 133–141.

Gurran, N. and Phibbs, P. (2013) Housing supply and urban planning reform: The recent Australian experience, 2003–2012. *International Journal of Housing Policy*, 13(4) pp. 381–407.

Gurran, N. and Phibbs, P. (2017) When tourists move in: How should urban planners respond to Airbnb? *Journal of the American Planning Association*, 83(1) pp. 80–92.

Heart Foundation (2004) *Healthy by Design: A Guide to Planning Environments for Active Living in Victoria*, Heart Foundation, Melbourne.

Heart Foundation (2018) *Healthy Active by Design*, Heart Foundation, Australia, www.healthyactivebydesign.com.au/ [Accessed 13 July 2018].

Hiscock, R., Kearns, A., MacIntyre, S. and Ellaway, A. (2001) Ontological security and psycho-social benefits from the home: Qualitative evidence on issues of tenure. *Housing, Theory and Society*, 18(1–2) pp. 50–66.

Howden-Chapman, P., Matheson, A., Crane, J., Viggers, H., Cunningham, M., Blakely, T., Cunningham, C., Woodward, A., Saville-Smith, K. and O'Dea, D. (2007) Effect of insulating existing houses on health inequality: Cluster randomised study in the community. *BMJ*, 334 p. 460.

Hulse, K., Pawson, H., Reynolds, M. and Herath, S. (2014) *Disadvantaged Places in Urban Australia: Analysing Socio-Economic Diversity and Housing Market Performance*, AHURI Final Report No. 225, Australian Housing and Urban Research Institute Limited, Melbourne.

Kearns, A., Hiscock, R., Ellaway, A. and McIntyre, S. (2000) 'Beyond four walls'. The psycho-social benefits of home: Evidence from West Central Scotland. *Housing Studies*, 15(3) pp. 387–410.

Kent, J. L. (2018) *Pole Position: Transport and Wellbeing in a Greenfield Estate*, A report for the Henry Halloran Trust, University of Sydney, Sydney, NSW.

Mallett, S., Bentley, R., Baker, E., Mason, K., Keys, D., Kolar, V. and Krnjacki, L. (2011) *Precarious Housing and Health Inequalities: What Are the Links?* Hanover Welfare Services, University of Melbourne, University of Adelaide, Melbourne City Mission, Australia.

Martin, C., Hulse, K., Pawson, H., Hayden, A., Kofner, S., Schwartz, A. and Stephens, M. (2018) *The Changing Institutions of Private Rental Housing: An International Review*, AHURI Final Report No. 292, Australian Housing and Urban Research Institute Limited, Melbourne.

Morris, A., Hulse, K. and Pawson, H. (2017) Long-term private renters: Perceptions of security and insecurity. *Journal of Sociology*, 53(3) pp. 653–669.

Nicholls, L., McCann, H., Strengers, Y. and Bosomworth, K. (2017) *Electricity Pricing, Heatwaves and Household Vulnerability in Australia*, Centre for Urban Research, RMIT, Melbourne.

Pawson, H., Martin, C., Flanagan, K. and Phillips, R. (2016) *Recent Housing Transfer Experience in Australia: Implications for Affordable Housing Industry Development*, AHURI Final Report No. 273, Australian Housing and Urban Research Institute, Melbourne.

Power, E. (2017) For renters, making housing more affordable is just the start, in Walton, J. ed., *Conversation Yearbook 2017: 50 Standout Articles from Australia's Top Thinkers*, Melbourne University Press, Melbourne.

Randolph, B., Troy, L., Milligan, V. and van den Nouwelant, R. (2018) *Paying for Affordable Housing in Different Market Contexts*, AHURI Final Report No. 293, Australian Housing and Urban Research Institute Limited, Melbourne.

UK Green Building Council (2016) *Health and Wellbeing in Homes*, UK Green Building Council, London.

Veitch, J., Bagley, S., Ball, K. and Salmon, J. (2006) Where do children usually play? A qualitative study of parents' perceptions of influences on children's active free-play. *Health and Place*, 12(4) pp. 383–393.

Waitt, G. R. and Farbotko, C. (2011) Residential air-conditioning and climate change: Voices of the vulnerable. *Health Promotion Journal of Australia*, 22(4) pp. 13–16.

Western Australian Planning Commission (2015) *Liveable Neighbourhoods*, Department of Planning, Perth.

Wilkins, R. (2017) *The Household, Income and Labour Dynamics in Australia Survey: Selected Findings from Waves 1 to 15*, Melbourne Institute, University of Melbourne, Melbourne.

Yardley, J., Sigal, R. J. and Kenny, G. P. (2011) Heat health planning: The importance of social and community factors. *Global Environmental Change*, 21(2) pp. 670–679.

Yates, J., Milligan, V., Berry, M., Burke, T., Gabriel, M., Pinnegar, S. and Randolph, B. (2007) *Housing Affordability: A 21st Century Problem*, AHURI Final Report no. 105, Australian Housing and Urban Research Institute Limited, Melbourne.

8 Public Open Spaces

Introduction

The importance of public open space provision in cities is recognised in United Nations Sustainable Development Goal 11.7, which, by the year 2030, aims to "provide universal access to safe, inclusive and accessible, green and public spaces, in particular for women and children, older persons and persons with disabilities" (United Nations 2015).

The need to prioritise the provision and maintenance of public open space in urban areas cannot be overemphasised. Public open spaces are a vital component of the city that, if managed properly, can promote many elements of human health. Public open spaces can host physical activity and community connections, and they can be spaces for growing fresh food. They are the lungs of an urban area that are so vital to the protection of biodiversity and mitigation of environmental risks. If public spaces are inadequate or not managed appropriately, urban life becomes private, opportunities to interact and be physically active are compromised, and the risk of a society that is isolated, sedentary and disjointed increases.

What Do We Mean by Public Open Spaces?

The term 'public open space' is an overarching concept. It encompasses a variety of spaces that are readily and, ideally, freely accessible to everyone, regardless of the size, design or physical features of the space. In particular, public open spaces have two distinct qualities. Firstly, they are the quintessentially democratic spaces of a city. This simply means that their allocation and maintenance prioritise equity. Use is not conditional on some kind of economic transaction, such as the need to pay an entry fee or purchase goods. Secondly, public open spaces have a special quality of being open-air, meaning they are spaces where contact with nature is more likely. They are often the spaces that green the city, supporting a standard of biodiversity and exposure to natural elements that would otherwise be missing.

There are many types of public open spaces. The term is used by government authorities in Australia to describe every different size of park, garden, reserve and waterway as well as the publicly owned forecourts, malls and squares scattered between buildings in urban areas. Public open spaces can be linear spaces that act as transport corridors. This includes walking and cycling networks and canals, creeks or rivers. They can be fitted out with a diverse array of facilities—from picnic pavilions and chess sets to ping-pong tables and all shapes and sizes of facilities for sitting and resting. They can be off-leash dog parks, community gardens, children's playgrounds, outdoor gyms or sculpture parks. Yet they are just as likely to be natural and uncultivated spaces—places for escape. Australian public open spaces include large tracts of relatively untamed regional parklands, iconic coastlines and areas of protected bushland known as National Parks. Of course, they also include Australia's world-famous beaches (see Box 8.1). Last but by no means least, Australia's public open spaces are the grounds and facilities that host our long tradition of participation and success in organised sports. Access to netball courts, rugby union, league, hockey, soccer and cricket grounds, as well as skate parks, velodromes and tennis courts, is a privilege that is taken for granted by many children growing up in Australia. Provision and maintenance of such facilities remain a high priority for Local government authorities.

Box 8.1   Australia's beaches and coastline

Because Australia's major cities are mostly located on the coast, the majority of Australians live close enough to a beach to ensure that a return trip can be comfortably accomplished within a day. With appropriate protection from the hot sun and other dangers such as powerful surf conditions, sharks, 'blue bottles' and jellyfish, a trip to the beach is a very Australian and generally very healthy day out. This is not least because it will usually include physical activity and connection with family, friends, community and nature as well as the calming presence of water. As public spaces, Australia's iconic beaches are therefore appealing and healthy environments that need to be protected both from the biophysical damages associated with climate change (including rising sea levels and the increased incidence of powerful and destructive surf events) and the ever-present pressure for privatisation of beach and coastal space. Unlike many countries around the world, Australia has generally resisted this pressure to privatise, and most of our beaches remain open to the public. In fact, our beaches are very democratic spaces—a source of national pride and a resource for the enjoyment of all.

The Interface Between Public and Private Spaces in Australia

The boundaries between what is public and private, open and enclosed, are shaped by a myriad of factors, including ownership, location, use and time of day or year. All of these variables can shift to ensure that what is public can become private and vice versa.

Not all publicly owned facilities are considered to be public open spaces. Indoor publicly owned spaces, such as schools, public hospitals and government offices, are not public open spaces because they are not accessible to all and are not characterised by the quality of being open-air. While transport networks, particularly footpaths and cycleways, are often considered public open spaces, whether a road space is public can depend on the mode used to traverse it. Driving a car on a public road, for example, is generally a private and enclosed act, whereas cycling along that same road is a more exposed way to travel that will most likely result in direct visual, verbal or aural connection with those around us. Public open spaces can also be ancillary to private uses. For example, a hospital may contain grounds that are publicly accessible and open for use by people not necessarily associated with the hospital's services. Similarly, private spaces can be ancillary to public spaces, such as an open air café located within the grounds of a large park.

The idea of semi-public spaces and ancillary uses leads us to question whether the definition of what is public/open space, as opposed to private/enclosed space, can be made with as much clarity as planners, policymakers and even the public generally assume. Private organisations are increasingly involved in creating, funding, managing or controlling public space. Places of retail trade and consumption are an interesting example in Australia (see Box 8.2). This push towards reliance on private management of public space is a global phenomenon that has evoked a rich body of scholarly work traversing disciplines as diverse as urban design, sociology, critical geography and property law. Often it is the proper management of this shifting interface between public and private ownership and use that can make an urban space convivial, appealing and, ultimately, healthy.

Box 8.2 The public/private space interface—retail trade as a case study

In a review of a controversial shopping centre development in Sydney in the mid-1990s, property lawyer Malcolm Voyce references the agora from ancient Greece as the first recorded notion of public open space in cities. Between the 18th and 8th Centuries BC, each city-state in Greece maintained an agora—initially as a place of civic gathering (much like the modern-day council chambers in Australia) but also as a place of commerce and trade. The agora provides confirmation of the fact places of trade have traditionally been conceptualised as public and democratic: "a place of pleasurable jostling, where citizens' bodies, words, actions and produce were all literally on mutual display, and where judgements, decisions and bargains were made" (Hartley 1992, pp. 29–30).

Unlike many European cities, Australia has never really established a tradition of regular public markets. This is likely the result of dispersed populations and the fact that our cities developed during the golden age of the automobile and the refrigerator, making a daily trip to and from a local market unnecessary. Until the 1950s, the inner central business districts of cities were the real hives of retail trade, with shopping opportunities in suburbs limited to high streets, often containing a butcher, greengrocer, bakery, fishmonger and perhaps a haberdashery or pharmacy. These open streets were, ostensibly, democratic public spaces. And while one might be expected to either make or browse for a purchase if entering an actual shop, the street itself was accessible to everyone at all times. To reinforce this accessibility, the street was often adorned with seating, trees and other public embellishments to encourage lingering, exchange and conviviality.

The extension of more comprehensive retail trade into Australia's suburbs strengthened after World War II. This was a boom provoked by suburbanisation, the availability of mass-produced consumer goods and economic stability. By the 1960s, the private car enabled cross-suburban travel, and several large department stores and chain speciality shops found welcoming premises in specially constructed 'big box' shopping centres (known in the United States as malls). Since their emergence, suburban shopping centres, and the question of whether they are public or private spaces, have attracted interest from academics and social commentators. Critics have derided their existence as perpetuating private car use, destroying local shopping strips and privatising what has traditionally been the public space of the market (Mitchell 1995; McGreevy 2016). Others point out that shopping centres are more open-access than other private uses and do contribute to some of the health benefits associated with public spaces, such as social interaction (see, for example, White et al. 2015). In Australia, there is evidence to support both claims. For some, the shopping centre provides a meeting place for friends, somewhere to go on a rainy day and somewhere that is reliably air-conditioned when the temperatures heat up in summer. Many shopping centres provide transport to and from the venue for the elderly and others without private car access. And perhaps most obviously related to health, mall walking is an increasingly popular activity in Australian shopping centres—again, providing a convivial place where physical activity can be undertaken in a climate-controlled and safe environment. Those making a case for a shift away from the big box shopping centre highlight the fact that shopping centres are designed to intercept, or filter, both visitors and retailers, using various techniques to exclude some while welcoming others. Shopping centres also have the legal capacity to exclude individuals and have been particularly criticised for their exclusion of minority groups such as the homeless and young people.

There are obviously positives and negatives to the cultural institution that has become the shopping centre in Australia's suburbs. As always with healthy planning, considerations of context must be at the heart of any evaluation of the effects of the privatisation of traditionally public retail spaces. Practices of operation, the design and the interface of the centre with its locality will differ from centre to centre, and as such, so will its impact on health. Of relevance to this chapter is that shopping centres are indicative of a trend in Australia and around the world towards the privatisation of the public—whether it be public space or services. This ostensibly neo-liberal approach has health implications, which are further discussed in Chapter 11—Reflections on Principles of Healthy Planning.

How Do Public and Open Spaces Influence Health?

The mechanisms underlying the links between public open space access and health are inevitably contextual and interconnected. For example, plentiful access to public open spaces is particularly important for encouraging physical activity for recreation as well as the incidental interactions critical to mental and physical health. Green and natural open spaces, in particular, are integral to the maintenance of biodiversity, which helps protect the planet's health. These spaces have the capacity to mitigate the urban heat island effect accompanying climate change—a function that will only increase in importance as our cities heat up. In addition to these more obvious links between public open space and health, we cannot deny that simply having spaces that are open, free to use and inherently natural in our urban areas is deeply soothing and foundational for human health.

Models have been proposed to capture these synergies. Swedish-based environmental psychologist Terry Hartig is widely considered a world expert on the importance of restorative spaces in cities. In 2014, he led an international team of similarly esteemed academics to propose four principal pathways through which public open spaces, and particularly natural spaces, can contribute to health: enhanced physical activity, greater social cohesion, stress reduction and improved air quality (Hartig et al. 2014). We use these pathways to draw out some of the links between public open spaces and health that are particularly relevant to both the planning and health challenges facing Australia.

Public Open Spaces and Physical Activity

The need for Australians to be more physically active has been described in detail in Chapter 4—Planning for Physical Activity. Public open space is a key component of built environments that encourage physical activity. This has been proven empirically by several Australian studies, including the landmark and longitudinal RESIDE study in Western Australia. This research found that people who take advantage of public open space are more likely to achieve recommended levels of physical activity. Components of this study also found that residents within 400 metres of a park were significantly more likely to partake in moderate to vigorous physical activity on a weekly basis (Hooper et al. 2018).

Most parts of Australia have a climate that enables outdoor recreation all year round, and the nation is well known for appreciating life spent outdoors. As a consequence, public open spaces are often relied upon for physical activity. For example, walking for recreation is the most common form of physical activity for Australian adults (Australian Bureau of Statistics [ABS] 2015). Public open space is an integral component of recreational walkability for several reasons. Firstly, the destinations that people walk to are frequently public open spaces. Secondly, public open space is a key element in diverse neighbourhoods. Parks, squares and water bodies provide an interesting backdrop to walk by, making this activity more appealing. Finally, and perhaps most importantly, recreational walking often occurs within public open spaces. The presence and maintenance of parks within a walkable distance of where people live and work can mean the difference between a walk that becomes a healthy habit and one that only happens when there is spare time to drive to the park.

Of course, walking is not the only physical activity occurring in Australia's public open spaces. Public recreational facilities, such as sports grounds, are particularly important for children's physical activity. Over 60% of the nation's children participate in outdoor organised sport such as netball, cricket, football and tennis (Australian Sports Commission 2016). This is primarily possible because of the grounds and courts that are reserved through land use planning and maintained by local authorities. Public open space is also a key component of children's improvised play, which occurs in any open space that is safe, interesting, close to home or school and well maintained. In short, the various public open spaces that punctuate our cities are the most accessible and obvious places for Australians to strengthen and renew their relationship with physical activity. Any attempt to increase physical activity in Australia must focus on providing equitable access to quality public open spaces across our urban areas.

Public Open Spaces and Social Interaction

The importance of incidental and planned social interactions for health is covered in Chapter 5—Planning for Social Interaction. Public open spaces are key to healthy social interactions because they are often the very places that host and encourage connection and engagement.

Some planners and scholars refer to public open spaces as 'third places', distinguishing them from other areas such as places of work, commerce or domesticity. They are the places in between the household and economic functions of modern life. Williams and Pocock (2010) argue that third places are fertile grounds for encouraging connected networks of community, not least because of their ability to promote incidental interactions. When we use the parks, trails, pedestrian malls and building forecourts that make up the public open space network, we are more likely to come into some contact with those around us. The more opportunities available for people to experience positive associations with those around them, no matter how minor, the greater the chance of developing tangible, lasting and caring connections, or at the very least a positive appraisal of our community and our city. In addition to hosting incidental social interactions, public open spaces are also important as the spaces that we often use to meet family and friends. The democratic nature of public open space ensures accessibility, providing a freely accessible venue for catch-ups, celebrations and other communal gatherings.

Public Open Spaces, Stress and Refuge

Rooted in the biophilia hypothesis (Wilson 1984), we know that there is an instinctive bond between human beings and other living systems. Again, this special relationship is covered in detail in Chapter 5—Planning for Social Interaction. As well as supporting physical activity and social connection, nature in cities has an intrinsic impact on health by providing spaces of refuge and distraction. This association was proved in an Australian context by a research team led by Takemi Sugiyama. Survey data from 1,895 residents of Adelaide revealed relationships between mental and physical health and perceived greenness in the environment. Among the research team's detailed conclusions, they found a significant relationship between greenness and mental health; however, recreational walking and social coherence accounted for only part of this association (Sugiyama et al. 2008).

Research confirms the Sugiyama findings time and time again. 'Building out' natural elements—including plants, animals and even the weather—is fundamentally detrimental to human health. International work includes a review of 50 articles examining the health benefits associated with mere visual contact with nature carried out by evolutionary biologists Bjørn Grinde and Grete Patil (2009). Australian public health researchers Mardi Townsend and Rona Weerasuriya also amassed a huge body of literature demonstrating the many direct benefits of green spaces and nature for health. This review, commissioned by Australia's National Depression Initiative, beyondblue, remains one of the most comprehensive and applied analyses of literature on the devastating mental health impacts of deprivation of contact with nature in urban areas (Townsend and Weerasuriya 2010).

What is it exactly about nature, greenery and openness that evokes feelings of refuge and distraction in modern life? In short, natural spaces allow us to escape—preferably to the extent where we can sense being somehow "in a different world" (Cooper Marcus and Sachs 2014, p. 28). While this might be a difficult sense to bestow through provision and design of a public square or building forecourt, it does suggest that our parks need to be sufficiently sized to enable us to experience a change— whether that be of scenery, use, design or atmosphere. We need to see, smell, hear and feel something different from the places of the city that promote stress. This sense of escape is heightened because of the fascination provided by natural things. Fascination provides distraction and a focus for techniques such as mindfulness and meditation. Open spaces, therefore, need to be interesting, incorporating natural elements to provide multiple objects of interest through flora, fauna, movement and light.

Places to Preserve

Public open spaces, particularly green spaces and waterways, are also the lungs of our city. They provide the corridors for flora and fauna to endure the demands of an urban environment and the biomass that absorbs greenhouse gas emissions. As well, green spaces improve microclimates and assist in reducing air pollution and urban runoff, which, in turn, results in cleaner waterways. Cooling the hot city, particularly in relation to the urban heat island, is another significant benefit that accrues from green space in our cities. These multiple (or co-) benefits are further elaborated in Chapter 3—Planning for the Health of the Planet.

Planning for Healthy Public Open Spaces in Australia

How can urban planning in Australia create and maintain healthy public open spaces? In evaluating thousands of public spaces around the world, not-for-profit organisation Project for Public Spaces identifies key components that interact to deliver thriving public open spaces (Project for Public Spaces 2018). These elements are as follows:

- Accessibility and linkages
- Sociability
- Uses and activities
- Comfort and image

The remainder of this chapter is inspired by the Project for Public Spaces framework, augmented by an additional focus on the distribution and management of these elements. This recognises that it is not only design and access that determine a healthy open space but also the amount of space provided throughout the city and its ongoing maintenance. Starting with this important element of distribution, we now progress to detail how each of these elements impacts health and conclude with some reflections on how we plan for these elements in Australia.

Healthy Public Open Space Distribution

Public open space distribution refers to the location, type and amount of public open space that is woven throughout an urban area. For public open spaces to facilitate physical activity, connection and rejuvenation, sufficient spaces of different types need to be provided. These spaces must be located close to the people who will use them. Similar principles apply to open spaces for environmental protection. However, proximity to people is not so much a key consideration as is the need to preserve specific types of biodiversity and geomorphology.

The question of how much public open space is required to support health dominates both research and practice on open space planning in Australia. There are numerous methods used to determine the optimal amount. They include providing space on the basis of population density or land mass. These quantitative indices are an obvious and useful starting point; however, best practice now recognises the need to balance qualitative assessments of needs, capacity, access and adaptability with quantitative standards. The following section proposes four guiding principles for qualitative evaluations of healthy public open space distribution.

Needs Analysis

One way to incorporate a qualitative component in distributing public open space is to analyse the needs of a locality. This takes account of demographic context and socio-economic variables as well as the existing built environment in which open spaces are situated. Different populations have varying needs. For example, areas with a high proportion of families with young children require more playgrounds and open spaces for improvised play as well as sports fields. Suburbs with a high concentration of elderly and retired people might be better served with trails for walking accompanied by plenty of seating areas to meet others. Analysing needs must be viewed as an ongoing process. Regular needs-based assessments of open space requirements enable planners to spot changing trends in demographics and recreational practices. For example, a recent review by the main Local government authority in inner Sydney, City of Sydney (2016), revealed that preferences for lunchtime sport in the central business district have shifted from organised team sports to more casual 'show up and play' games. Games such as '6-a-side soccer', 'touch football' and 'Oztag' require half fields, and their promotion is a great opportunity to encourage more people to be physically active in less space. If the Local Council had overlooked this trend and continued to provide full-sized fields, it may have missed a valuable opportunity to encourage physical activity and interactions within the local area.

The question then arises about the best way to assess the needs of a particular community or urban area. Australian guidelines for public open space planning generally recommend community consultation to ascertain needs. Although this should not be the sole source of information, it is an indispensable one. Users can be consulted about their 'level of interest' in certain activities or requested to make direct suggestions for facilities they would like to see provided. Language is important here, and good practice shows the benefits of investigating what future users might need in order to actually use a space. This nuanced shift in the mode of enquiry enables the user to speak within the context of their lifestyle as well as their built environment. For example, while a user might express interest in access to a community garden, to ensure it is used, they might also need the garden to be located within walkable distance of a bus stop. By leaving the question 'what do you need?' open-ended, the provider is given the opportunity to plan public open space that is truly responsive to context. It is then, importantly, likely to be effective in promoting health. Of course, open-ended consultation processes are inevitably more resource-intensive to analyse. However, resources invested in a comprehensive needs analysis might save the monumental waste associated with provision of unwanted spaces. Such consultative needs assessments must also be accompanied by several other sources of data, including a land use assessment of existing provisions and socio-economic and demographic data. Increasingly, in Australia, public health authorities are asked to provide health data in the process of planning for public open space. We suggest that this is a perfect entry point for ongoing collaboration between health and planning professionals.

Equitable Access and Outcomes

Although needs can be assessed in different ways, such an analysis should be motivated by equitable access aspirations. Regardless of an individual's residential location or socio-economic background, they should enjoy access to well-maintained public open space across the city. Several recent studies in Australia, however, clearly show deficiencies here. For example, a study of 1,500 parks in Melbourne found that parks located in suburbs of relatively socio-economically disadvantaged communities had poorer quality and fewer facilities, including trees, shade, water features, walking paths, lighting and signage (Crawford et al. 2008). Another more recent quantitative evaluation of green open space provision against socio-economic variables found that there were fewer green open spaces available in poorer areas across all Australian capital cities (Astell-Burt et al. 2014). While these studies reveal some quite obvious equity gaps in the provision of open space, there is also evidence of more subtle signs of inequity in our approach to public open space distribution. For example, many of our major city and regional parks can only be accessed by private car, rendering their use by those without a car or a driver's license problematic.

Adaptability

Adaptability is another useful principle to apply in planning public open space for health. Planners, including those planning for healthy built environments, often advocate flexibility and multipurpose use as a way to maximise the distribution of uses across an urban area. This is particularly important in areas of rapid population growth and densification, where there is inevitably an ever-dwindling amount of space available for public use. This can be as simple as providing spaces for sitting along a walking trail or locating children's play spaces next to outdoor gyms. We do, however, cite two caveats to multifunctional public open space provision in the Australian context. Firstly, multiuse spaces should not rely on a private use to make them work. For example, a coffee cart within a park might do well to attract people to the facility; however, park users should not feel as though they have to make a purchase to enjoy the space. As discussed above, the privatisation of uses in public open space is an increasingly popular trend in Australia, and this is a practice that requires careful monitoring. Secondly, a public open space cannot be all things to all people, and for some, the most appealing space might be one that is relatively sparse and reliably quiet. Accordingly, there is a need to balance the provision of multiple uses against the needs of those simply seeking a place for time out.

Capacity to Maintain and Manage

Decisions on public open space distribution need to be made in the context of the governing authority's capacity to manage the use over the long-term. To become attached to a space, people need to feel it has a sense of permanency, and it needs to be well maintained. Consistent management of the space and a physically and administratively networked approach to public open space maintenance are essential requirements of planning for healthy public open space. These are tasks that require integration of regional and local perspectives. Failure to allocate responsibility for public open space networks leaves them vulnerable to development for other purposes.

The Distribution of Open Space in Australia

Knowing that best-practice open space distribution incorporates consideration of community needs, equity, adaptability, capacity and existing and future networks, how are these decisions made in Australia? The distribution of public open space is managed differently in each Australian State and across all scales of government. Local Councils have primary responsibility for the types of spaces provided. Councils generally maintain some form of typology to classify their public open space assets for management. These are basically inventories of space. Typically, classification schemas are based upon the size of the space, its deemed function and geographic location and the types of facilities present. State authorities also influence the distribution of public open space through strategic planning functions, the issuance of guidance to Local government and involvement in major infrastructure and urban development projects. While the Federal government is generally absent from discussions of public open space, its involvement in major infrastructure funding ensures participation in discussions of public open space distribution from time to time. A variety of other authorities are involved in public open space provision. For example, individual sporting bodies recommend required dimensions and equipment for particular sports. These various guidelines are then applied across spaces that are managed by all jurisdictions, from Local to State and Federal.

Although different levels of government take responsibility for public open space distribution, common to all is that decisions around spaces and facilities in Australia are inevitably subject to political, economic and cultural scrutiny. As a use primarily for the public good rather than the profit of any one particular individual or the private sector, the protection of public open space across our urban areas is subject to intense competition and debate. This competition is only increasing as densities in our urban areas increase (see Box 8.3). The way we distribute public open space is also constrained by the various historical legacies that have shaped Australian urban areas. Again, we see that context, both past and present, must be a key consideration when looking at links between the built environment and health.

Box 8.3   Density and public open space in Australia

Increased densities in Australian cities will require greater provision of public open space; however, it is not quite that simple (Byrne et al. 2010). People living in apartments and townhouses have less access to private open space, and therefore will tend to live more of their outdoor lives within the public realm. Some of the activities that Australians have taken for granted to date—keeping a pet, playing backyard cricket with the kids or hosting a BBQ—inevitably spill out into public open spaces, and it is the responsibility of Australia's planners to ensure that this happens in a convivial way.

If there is sufficient and well-maintained public open space, the drift of traditionally private practices into public spaces can ignite the health-promoting elements of a convivial place. When spaces are in short supply, inappropriately designed or poorly managed, they become spaces of tension that feel unsafe and unappealing. The message is that it has never been more important in Australia for planners to consider the shifting needs of the population when determining the types and amounts of open space required. We must account for our transitioning culture.

Perhaps it is the highly politicised nature of public open space provision that has reinforced Australian planning's ongoing attachment to quantitative standards for public open space distribution. A clear quantifiable requirement is nearly always defensible in the face of competition for space more generally. Regardless, various analyses of planning for public open space in Australia reveal not only an over-reliance on quantitative standards but also little evidence-based rationale for the standards used. For example, up until the turn of the century, the most common measurement for the provision of public open space in Australia was 2.83 hectares per 1,000 people. A very interesting historical review conducted by Veal (2013) reveals that this standard is derived from the British '7 acres per 1,000' standard from the early 1900s, and that "no one ever really asked if this UK standard was appropriate; it was simply adopted. . . .

Even in the early '70s when the first review of open space was carried out, the then State Planning Authority didn't query this standard and simply converted it to metric" (Shiels 1989, p. 12).

Although the majority of plans for public open space in Australia now advocate the benefit of a needs-based, context-sensitive approach to the distribution of space, specific numerical indicators and targets are still quoted regularly in plans and practice. An example is the New South Wales' *Recreation and Open Space Planning Guidelines for Local Government* (Department of Planning 2010b), which provides default standards for open space planning. These include 9% of site area for local and district level open space provision and 15% for regional open space provision. As established above, quantitative standards are a relatively unsophisticated approach to public open space provision, particularly this kind of 'fixed provision' standard based on quantities such as the amount of land or population to be served by the space. Even though new technologies using big data are emerging to increase the ease and speed at which public open spaces can be quantified, nothing compares to the rich data collected when the researcher actually visits and experiences the site first hand.

Accessibility and Linkages

We have already noted above that public open spaces come in a variety of shapes and sizes and are used for many different activities. Planning these diverse spaces for health requires that they are considered as a network of interconnected elements, rather than a disparate collection of land parcels. This simply means looking at the way people will travel to, through, around and from public open spaces as well as the way spaces are positioned, or linked, to other uses. This networked perspective is important for the health-promoting capacity of public open space for several reasons.

Firstly, strategic positioning of public open space within the context of other uses enhances the likelihood that people will be able to access spaces by active modes. This means that spaces are located within walking distance of homes, jobs and schools. Living and working in close proximity to public open space enhances the ease of access and appeal of spaces, positioning the space as a destination for walking.

Secondly, consideration of public open space as a network of linkages reveals the array of smaller spaces that exist between uses, such as linear parkways, malls, forecourts, laneways and squares. Valuing joined-up spaces as open space more broadly bestows a sense of synergy on the built environment by bringing together its constituent parts. Such synergy enhances the appeal of the space and encourages people to be out and about in their built environment. This can be as simple as maintaining a footpath, or providing lighting or seating in a square, or as radical as painting the blank walls of a laneway with a mural. A network approach enables a more realistic inventory of what is existing within an urban area as well as the ability to spot gaps where additional space of a certain type might be required. Networks of public open space can also be used to alleviate open space deficits by maximising connections and crossing points to create a larger catchment area.

Thirdly, links between open spaces have the capacity to host healthy activities in their own right. Walking or cycling through a network of pathways connecting parks, squares and plazas provides an additional option for physical activity, encouraging people to be out and about, exploring their built environment. Linked and linear open spaces are also imperative for protecting biodiversity corridors. The use of links for individual healthy practices, such as walking and cycling, needs to be balanced against this important environmental consideration.

While Australia's planners are increasingly recognising the need to plan for networks of open space, this is a relatively new approach (see the Sydney case study in Box 8.4). Our nation's open spaces are managed by multiple agencies operating at very different scales, often with conflicting stakeholder interests. Room remains for regional coordination of public open space provision to ensure that resources are maximised, provision is contextualised and gaps in delivery in lower socio-economic areas are closed. The need for open space connectivity is discussed below.

Box 8.4 Green spaces in Australia's largest city, Sydney

This brief review of green space planning in Australia's largest city, Sydney, demonstrates the way history and politics determine green open space planning.

Proclamations of recreation lands by Colonial Governors were the first examples of parks in Sydney. Following the English tradition of a town common, 'the Common' (later Hyde Park) was proclaimed by Governor Macquarie in 1810, with a second common of 1,000 acres (now Centennial Park and Moore Park) dedicated in 1811. As the city grew, lobbyists placed increasing pressure on the Government to reserve areas for open space. The funds accompanying the New South Wales *Land for Public Purposes Acquisition Act of 1880* enabled the Government to resume land for recreation grounds. Local authorities were delegated managerial responsibility for open space, and many new parks were proclaimed, mostly in middle- to high-income suburbs. In addition, pocket parks were established on land deemed unfit for development.

During this time, there was no overarching metropolitan strategy guiding the development of land or green space in Sydney. This changed in 1948 with the release of Sydney's first strategic plan, the *County of Cumberland Planning Scheme for Sydney* (1948), which included a green belt. This comprised a strip of open country linking Ku-ring-gai Chase National Park in the north with the Royal National Park in the south. Continual pressure for exemptions allowing development on the green belt, combined with the promotion of linear expansion and highway development to cope with population growth, saw the green belt much diminished in the subsequent 1968 *Sydney Regional Outline Plan*. The importance of green space has since fluctuated in recent metropolitan plans. 'Parks and Public Places' were included as one of seven key strategic areas in the *City of Cities Plan* (2005), whereas the *Metropolitan Plan for Sydney 2036* (2010a) had no objectives specifically related to open space. *A Plan for Growing Sydney* (2014) announced the creation of a city wide 'Green Grid', an interconnected network of open space and walking tracks, as part of its goal to create "a great place to live with communities that are strong, healthy and well connected" (Department of Planning and Environment 2014, p. 80). Sydney has grown during a time when open space has been highly valued, resulting in the reservation of larger areas of green space, such as national parks, foreshore reserves and regional recreation areas, including Penrith Lakes, Western Sydney Parklands, Bicentennial Park, Hyde Park, Centennial Park and Moore Park. However, the distribution of green space at the local scale is uneven. The objectives of the proposed Green Grid would help to redress some of this imbalance, but ongoing funding for this project is a concern. The Greater Sydney Commission identifies established programs (such as the Metropolitan Green Space Program and the Restoration and Rehabilitation Program, which already provide grants for capital works improvements for existing green spaces) and development contributions as possible sources of funding. However, no new streams of funding have been announced to accompany the implementation of the Green Grid.

The Sociability of Public Open Spaces

We often assume that a successful and healthy public open space is one that is well frequented, busy and somehow iconic. In arguing for the retention or provision of public open space, Australian planners often determine the value, or success, of a space by the number of people that might use it to socialise. However, not all public open spaces need to be overly populated or visually striking to be health-promoting. Sometimes the most cherished, restorative and appealing spaces are quiet, secluded and unassuming. When sufficient public open space is provided and those spaces are well managed, safe, connected and tailored to place, a successful open space need only convey a sense that it is respected and appreciated. This can mean that the space is clean, with facilities in working order. Or, for wild spaces, it might mean that it is protected, enabling the space to grow and shape its own natural position within the biosphere. We therefore translate the Project for Public Spaces attention to sociability of a space to mean not that it is busy and popular, but rather that it has a sense of vitality and is valued. This means that the space is *part of a society*, and that those planning, managing and using the wider built environment consistently deem the space worthy of retention. Sociability is a prerequisite for a space to promote health. If a space is not valued by those who own, manage and use it, it cannot fulfil its health-promoting potential, whether that be for physical activity or social interaction or as a space of nature—quiet and soothing.

Uses and Activities, Safety and Comfort

A key theme in this chapter has been that the mere presence of public open space does not guarantee its ability to promote health. Spaces need to be *actually used* if their health-promoting potential is to be maximised. Once we know the type of space to provide and where to provide it, how can we design and manage it to encourage use? Here are some suggestions.

People are drawn to spaces where they feel comfortable. This may not be a sense of physical comfort. While the provision of choices for people to sit where they want to sit is an undeniable component of the spaces that are well used, other types of public open space, such as outdoor gyms, trails for brisk walking or running and even community gardens, might not necessarily be physically comfortable during use. But to encourage use, they do need to promote a sense of belonging and sociability that reassures the user they are safe.

In terms of safety from crime, planners will often reference the concept of Crime Prevention Through Environmental Design (CPTED). We discuss this concept in detail in Chapter 5—Planning for Social Interaction. There are many links between built environments for crime prevention and those that support health. In the context of making public open spaces safe, the best defence is in enabling and encouraging regular use. This in turn supports surveillance and a sense of ownership and pride in the space.

In addition to the principles of CPTED, there are several other components of comfortable spaces that are well within the remit of healthy planning. The provision of the simplest of signage, for example, can ensure that people know how to behave in a space, which in turn promotes the harmonious use of that space. This might include ensuring that shared pathways are well marked and, where possible, separated, providing directional signage along walking trails or providing clear instructions for when and how to access a community garden. Providing a booking system for facilities that can be used by only one party at a time (such as tennis courts, cricket nets and in-demand picnic spots) will reduce tensions during peak periods. These initiatives will become even more important in areas where the population is growing and space is shrinking. The increased use of web-based apps for providing on-demand and real-time updates of the types and conditions of different public open spaces, including how busy they are, is a fruitful avenue for the future.

Finally, open spaces for health need to provide creature comforts and cover the basics of design safety for the prevention of accidents and protection from the elements. Facilities such as clean public toilets and drinking fountains (sometimes called 'bubblers' in Australia) can mean a neighbourhood park becomes an afternoon-long favourite, rather than a place that needs to be abandoned when nature calls. Shade sails over playground equipment provide some protection from the harsh Australian sun, ensuring that the benefits of outdoor physical activity are not eroded by the risk of skin cancer. There is a series of Australian Standards that cover the design of facilities such as playgrounds and other components of the public realm. *Australian Standard 4685* is the primary standard and a great place to start if detailed design advice is required.

Conclusion

Public open spaces are the lungs and lifeblood of Australia's urban areas. They are the spaces where we interact and learn to accommodate and appreciate diversity. They are democratic spaces where physical activity and time out are free of charge. While public open spaces alone do not make a healthy built environment, it is difficult to imagine a liveable city devoid of open space.

This chapter has focused on several key health benefits associated with public open space, placing particular emphasis on its restorative functions. Australians have traditionally conceptualised the outdoor components of urban areas as relatively private, symbolised by the distinct appreciation of owning a backyard, where rituals such as cricket and BBQs are played out. Yet cultural and urban changes are shifting this way of thinking about open spaces. As our cities grow and densify, the provision of public open spaces of adequate quality and quantity will be key. These are the spaces that will give new and changing communities the opportunity to connect, and our biophysical environment the chance to absorb the impacts of urban life.

References

Astell-Burt, T., Feng, X., Mavoa, S., Badland, H. M. and Giles-Corti, B. (2014) Do low-income neighbourhoods have the least green space? A cross-sectional study of Australia's most populous cities. *BMC Public Health*, 14 p. 292.

Australian Bureau of Statistics (2015) *Participation in Sport and Physical Recreation, Australia, 2013–2014*, Cat. no. 4177.0, Australian Bureau of Statistics, Canberra.

Australian Sports Commission (2016) *AusPlay: Participation Data for the Sport Sector*, Australian Government, Canberra.

Byrne, J., Sipe, N. and Searle, G. (2010) Green around the gills? The challenge of density for urban greenspace planning in SEQ. *Australian Planner*, 47(3) pp. 162–177.

City of Sydney (2016) *Open Space, Sports and Recreation Needs Study 2016, Volume 1: The Strategy*, City of Sydney, Sydney, NSW.

Cooper Marcus, C. and Sachs, N. (2014) *Therapeutic Landscapes: An Evidenced Based Approach to Designinghealing Gardens and Restorative Outdoor Spaces*. Wiley, New Jersey.

Crawford, D., Timperio, A., Giles-Corti, B., Ball, K., Hume, C., Roberts, R., Andrianopoulos, N. and Salmon, J. (2008) Do features of public open spaces vary according to neighbourhood socio-economic status? *Health and Place*, 14(4) pp. 889–893.

Cumberland County Council (1948) *County of Cumberland Planning Scheme Report*, Cumberland County Council, Sydney, NSW.

Department of Planning (2005) *City of Cities–A Plan for Sydney's Future*, NSW Government, Sydney, NSW.

Department of Planning (2010a) *Metropolitan Plan for Sydney 2036*, NSW Government, Sydney, NSW.

Department of Planning (2010b) *Recreation and Open Space Planning Guidelines for Local Government*, NSW Department of Planning, Sydney, NSW.

Department of Planning and Environment (2014) *A Plan for Growing Sydney*, NSW Government, Sydney, NSW.

Grinde, B. and Patil, G. G. (2009) Biophilia: Does visual contact with nature impact on health and well-being? *International Journal of Environmental Research and Public Health*, 6(9) pp. 2332–2343.

Hartig, T., Mitchell, R., de Vries, S. and Frumkin, H. (2014) Nature and health. *Annual Review of Public Health*, 35(1) pp. 207–228.

Hartley, J. (1992) *The Politics of Pictures: The Creation of the Public in the Age of Popular Media*, Routledge, London.

Hooper, P., Boruff, B., Beesley, B., Badland, H. and Giles-Corti, B. (2018) Testing spatial measures of public open space planning standards with walking and physical activity health outcomes: Findings from the Australian national liveability study. *Landscape and Urban Planning*, 171 pp. 57–67.

McGreevy, M. (2016) The economic and employment impacts of shopping mall developments on regional and peri-urban Australian towns. *Australasian Journal of Regional Studies*, 22(3) pp. 402–434.

Mitchell, D. (1995) The end of public space? People's Park, definitions of the public, and democracy. *Annals of the Association of American Geographers*, 85(1) pp. 108–133.

Project for Public Spaces (2018) *Resource Articles–Placemaking* 101, www.pps. org/reference/reference-categories/placemaking-tools/ [Accessed 28 June 2018].

Shiels, G. (1989) More quality, less quantity in open space planning. *Australian Parks and Recreation*, 25(1) pp. 12–14.

State Planning Authority (1968) *Sydney Regional Outline Plan*, NSW Government, Sydney, NSW.

Sugiyama, T., Leslie, E., Giles-Corti, B. and Owen, N. (2008) Associations of neighbourhood greenness with physical and mental health: Do walking, social coherence and local social interaction explain the relationships? *Journal of Epidemiology and Community Health*, 62(5) p. e9.

Townsend, M. and Weerasuriya, R. (2010) *Beyond Blue to Green: The Benefits of Contact with Nature for Mental Health and Well-Being*, Beyond Blue Limited, Melbourne.

United Nations (2015) *Transforming Our World: The 2030 Agenda for Sustainable Development*, Department of Economic and Social Affairs, New York.

Veal, A. J. (2013) Open space planning standards in Australia: In search of origins. *Australian Planner*, 50(3) pp. 224–232.

White, R., Toohey, J. A. and Asquith, N. (2015) Seniors in shopping centres. *Journal of Sociology*, 51(3) pp. 582–595.

Williams, P. and Pocock, B. (2010) Building 'community' for different stages of life: Physical and social infrastructure in master planned communities. *Community, Work and Family*, 13(1) pp. 71–87.

Wilson, E. O. (1984) *Biophilia*, Harvard University Press, Cambridge, MA.

9 Transport, Access and Health

Introduction

This chapter is about planning for healthy transport in Australian urban areas. Australia is a vast land mass. While predominantly clustered around the coast, our cities and towns are separated by relatively large expanses. Even within our urban areas, lower densities translate into long distances between uses, which, for some, makes lengthy travel times an inevitability.

The way we travel can have both negative and positive effects on health, depending on the structure and function of the transport network. In this chapter, we provide a way forward for a healthy transport system in Australia. Our recommendations are underpinned by a key goal for transport in Australia: to transition away from the harms of private car use while still enabling equitable access. We start with a general overview of the links between transport and health.

How Does Transport Influence Health?

There are countless links between transport and health. Most obvious are the direct health consequences of transport modes, including impacts on respiratory health and bodily injury and death associated with transport-related accidents. There are also less obvious health consequences, however, associated with transport's primary role: to enable access to the jobs, family, friends, healthy food, open space and spaces of care that support a healthy lifestyle.

When looking at the impacts of transport on health in Australia, we first need to acknowledge the place of the private car. In transport research, car use is often positioned as being a dominant, or 'hegemonic', transport system. For a number of historical, cultural and structural reasons, this is certainly true in Australia. Private road vehicles currently account for 87% of aggregate personal travel in urban areas, and Australia has one of the highest car ownership rates in the world (Bureau of Infrastructure, Transport and Regional Economics [BITRE] 2015). Cars in Australia remain closely linked to notions of individual consumption, economic production and cultural legitimisation as well as personal freedom, social status, reliability and comfort. This means that the car has a special place, not only in the way Australians travel but also in our national culture.

Reflecting this historical attachment, the dominance of the car is cemented, quite literally, in the structure of Australian cities. This is because cars became popular and accessible at the same time the nation's cities were growing. Throughout the long boom of the 1950s and 1960s, suburbs were built on the assumption that most new households would have a car. As a result, our cities today are low-density, with long distances separating uses. Our public transport systems are also relatively underdeveloped and struggle to bridge the distances associated with our sprawling cities. Other alternatives, such as walking and cycling, are marginalised, not only by insufficient infrastructure but also because the distances between uses in our cities are too great to cover by bike or on foot. As a result, most people in Australia today either prefer, or are forced, to depend on the car. This sense of dependence further legitimises car use as the cultural norm, and the car has become the standard of comfort, flexibility and autonomy expected in Australia. This is a reinforcing cycle, often referred to as the 'cycle of automobility' (see Figure 9.1).

Because Australian cities and lifestyles are so conditioned by the car, many of the links between the nation's transport and health are related to car use. The discussion that follows takes from this and features car use as problematic for, but also supportive of, health in Australia.

Transport-Related Collisions and Injuries

Traditionally, transport-related health research has focused on acute morbidity and mortality from transport accidents. In 2016, road accidents in Australia were responsible for 1,295 fatalities, equating to 5.37 road accident fatalities per 100,000 people (BITRE 2017). Less information exists about those seriously injured; however, it is estimated that 20 people are seriously injured for every recorded road death in Australia. The health impact of road accidents extends well beyond acute and physical injury. The long-term psychological effects of car accidents include post-traumatic stress disorder and other psychiatric conditions, which the World Health Organization (WHO) estimates affect up to 25% of survivors of serious accidents (WHO 2000). There are also broader impacts for families who lose loved ones or have to live with the consequences of disability and, for the nation as a whole, the loss of productivity. Furthermore, the car does not only pose injury risk to its drivers and passengers. The physical risks associated with walking are primarily a result of the need to share space with the car. Across the spectrum of severity, cycling

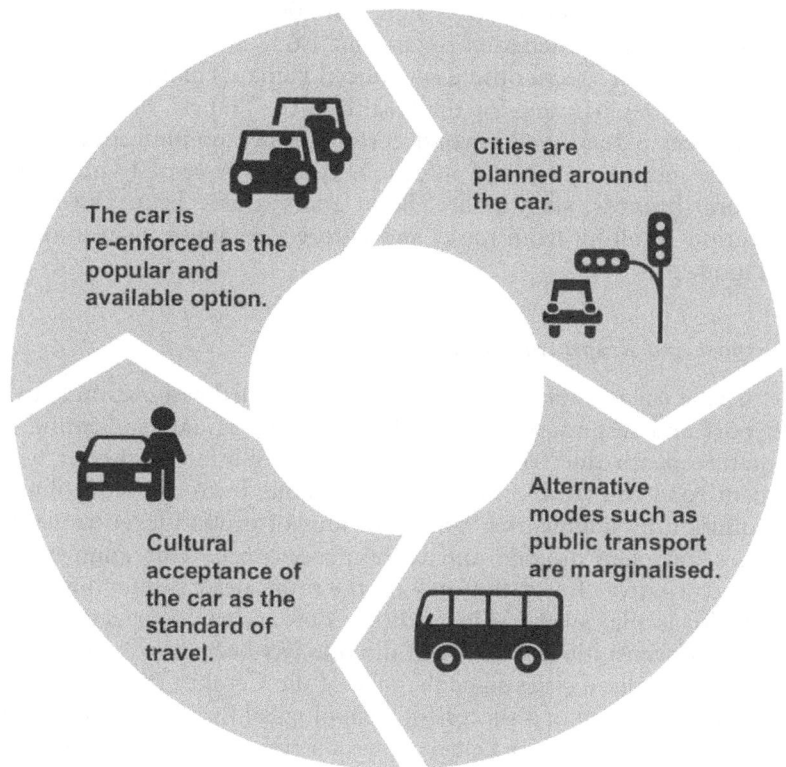

Figure 9.1 The cycle of automobility

Source: Adapted from Victoria Transport Policy Institute 2018

accidents are actually less likely to involve a car; however, cars are almost always implicated in cycling accidents where there is a fatality (Centre for Accident Research and Road Safety Queensland 2012).

Transport and Climate Change

Carbon dioxide is an air pollutant generated by the combustion of fuel and associated with car use. It does not have direct health effects at the very minimal concentrations occurring in the ambient environment (WHO 2000). It is, however, the main greenhouse gas causing global warming (Banister 2011) and as such indirectly contributes to the global health impact of climate change (Hickman et al. 2010). Transport contributes to around 13% of Australia's net greenhouse gas emissions, of which private cars are the main source (Climate Council 2017).

Transport emissions are also one of the strongest sources of emissions growth in Australia, being 35% higher in 2009 than in 1990. On average, emissions have increased by around 1.6% annually. The resultant health impacts of greenhouse gas–induced climate change are extensive (see Chapter 3—Planning for the Health of the Planet). In short, health consequences extend well beyond chronic, non-communicable diseases to include increasing rates of infectious disease, increased vulnerability to natural hazards, such as fire, flood and extreme heat, and societal dislocation resulting from rapid and enforced changes in location and livelihood.

Transport and Respiratory Illness

The private car is implicated in the well-researched association between transport and respiratory disease. Indeed, there is data indicating that premature death due to vehicle-related air pollution is similar to the accident road toll (Robinson 2005). Emissions from cars contribute to air pollution by augmenting concentrations of ground-level ozone, particulates, nitrogen dioxide and carbon monoxide. This augmentation can have negative effects, not only on the respiratory system but also on the cardiovascular system. On a positive note, research suggests that the ambient concentration of nitrogen dioxide has been slowly declining in many industrialised cities since the turn of the Century (Kjellstrom et al. 2002). This is a case of a successful technological fix. The mandatory use of catalytic converters for vehicle emission reduction was introduced in Australia in 1985, ameliorating some of the adverse impact of cars on respiratory health.

Transport and Physical Activity

Physical inactivity is a health risk factor for many Australians. In Chapter 4—Planning for Physical Activity—we outlined how active transport is a great opportunity to incorporate physical activity into day-to-day life. There are several ways, however, that Australia's transport systems and urban structures de-prioritise active transport modes. Firstly, the dominance of the private car hinders opportunities for those who prefer to travel by active modes, often replacing or compromising essential infrastructure such as footpaths and bike paths. The popularity of the car also detracts from the critical mass required to justify investment in public transport infrastructure. Further, land dedicated to car-related infrastructure, including land for parking, is land that cannot generally be used for recreational physical activity. Finally, the noise and air pollution associated with car transport has the potential to detract from the provision of pleasant recreational environments.

Transport, Stress and Community

A less obvious link between transport and health is the way our transport practices are implicated in the rush and busyness that characterise modern life. In Chapter 11—Reflections on Principles of Healthy Planning—we advocate the need to 'slow down' as a key health issue in Australia. It seems that, as a nation, we increasingly pack our schedules full of activities, fitting things in around work, family, friends and other commitments. The private car is pivotal here. It is the autonomous mobility afforded by the car that enables the accomplishment of multiple daily activities across Australia's relatively dispersed cities. In this way, private car use can be linked to the stress associated with mental illnesses such as anxiety and depression. There are several other ways transport is related to stress. Studies have shown that the physical restriction of being stuck in traffic or packed into an overcrowded train increases blood pressure and induces sensations of frustration. Research has also linked long commutes with decreased wellbeing (see Milner et al. 2017 for an Australian review) and traffic noise with nervousness, hearing impairment and depression. Through their ability to transform streets into depersonalised places of danger, noise and rush, cars, and the roads required for them, have also been associated with the dispersion of community fabric and community cohesion. Famous planning observer Jane Jacobs identified cars as "powerful and insistent instruments of city destruction" (Jacobs 1961, p. 352). This encroachment of the car into everyday spaces of connection—and the resultant scattering of community—is another tangible risk factor for various types of mental illness, including anxiety and depression (Nguyen 2010).

Transport and Equity

Transport research embraces not only the ability to travel but also the impacts of immobility or lack of access to transport. The inability to travel is increasingly explored as a component of social inequality, which is closely linked to health. Kaufmann et al. (2004) coined the term 'motility' to describe this particular type of social disparity. As with many public health issues, the negative health effects of transport practices, particularly the prevalence of the private car, are disproportionately borne by vulnerable populations. Although cars are extremely popular in Australia, car ownership and use are not an option for everyone. The frail elderly, visually impaired and financially stressed are all examples of groups excluded from the access provided by the car. The increasing complexity of getting a driver's license and the financial burden of maintaining a car have meant that many young Australians are not able (or willing) to buy into automobility as easily as has been the case in the past. And because Australian cities are designed around the assumption of everyone having access to a private car (the 'cycle of automobility' in Figure 9.1), access opportunities for these groups are constrained.

An Alternative View on the Links Between the Private Car and Health

Although often implicated in poor health outcomes, there are many reasons why cars also support human health in Australia. In cities that are sprawling, with long distances between uses and very little alternative transport provision, access to a car is often essential for getting to places of employment and different services and for visiting family and friends and participating in a range of activities. For most Australians, a car is a necessary, and often unquestioned, acquisition for participation in society.

Although rarely acknowledged in the active transport literature, it is also undeniable that, for many, cars bring a sense of individual comfort, autonomy and convenience. They provide shelter from the weather, enable access to multiple destinations and opportunities and free us from timetables. Private cars, in car-dependent nations such as Australia, are also important for practices of care, both for the self and others. Cars enable children to travel to school safely, the elderly to attend medical appointments, companion animals to visit the vet and others to visit loved ones in times of need. Cars are also spaces that are relatively private and inherently personal. For many people, driving a car is an opportunity for time out. The comfortable, air-conditioned, soundproofed and personalised interior of the car provides a relative cocoon from the world around us (Kent 2014b, Kent 2014c). Finally, cars in Australia are places where cultural rituals such as the family holiday, the school drop-off and the first date are lived out (Miller 2001). In the trend towards houses where children are often partitioned away from adults, the car provides a rare space where families are forced to be together.

So, What Exactly Is Healthy Transport in Australia?

Healthy built environment professionals often discuss active and public transport modes as the pinnacles of healthy transport. Walking and cycling certainly have benefits for health. They encourage physical activity and social interaction and can be a prompt to slow down our speeded-up, stressed out lives. Similarly, public transport can also encourage physical activity and interaction, not least because a public transport trip usually starts and finishes on foot or by bike. Cars are usually positioned at the opposite end of the spectrum of healthy transport, implicated in global harms, such as climate change and inequity, and associated with traffic congestion, physical inactivity and a detachment from life on the street. The review above, however, suggests that conceptualising 'healthy transport' is not as straightforward as positioning active and public transport against private car use. Firstly, there are many modes with health impacts that are in between the two. These are missed by this overly simplistic dichotomy. Emergent ways of sharing cars and combining modes are blurring the lines between active and other transport (Kent 2014a). Online technologies are opening up an approach that is flexible, on demand and multimodal. Secondly, as we have already discussed, for many in Australia, the car is still an important tool in maintaining a healthy and connected lifestyle both for ourselves and the people for whom we care. The key point is that a health-promoting transport system may not actually be one that is dominated by any one particular way of travelling. Instead, it will be a system that provides equitable access to transport options that can accommodate the complex needs and desires of modern life while minimising harms.

Planning for Healthy Transport in Australia

Our review of the health impacts of transport suggests that creating a healthy transport network in Australia will be a complex balancing act. It requires initiatives to temper the negative impacts of private car use and encourage alternative transport modes while still enabling access to all the things that make a happy, connected and healthy life. This demands acknowledgement of just how car-dependent our cities and lives are. As mentioned above, Australia's cities and towns have grown up in the era of the private car, and as such pursuit of some kind of 'no car' urban utopia is impractical. Once this fact and its implications are recognised, we can move forward with practical and effective ways to 'tame' the private car in Australia (Kent 2014b, p. 114).

The Importance of Urban Fabrics

A useful concept in transport planning, and one developed by influential Australian transport planners Peter Newman and Jeff Kenworthy (together with Leo Kosonen from Finland), is the theory of urban fabrics (Newman and Kenworthy 2015). This theory—or schema—simply proposes that there are three main types of urban fabrics that can be characterised by the way people travel within and around them. They are walking urban fabrics, public transport urban fabrics and private car urban fabrics. We consider that 'walking urban fabrics' is more usefully termed 'active transport urban fabrics'. This broader conceptualisation recognises that cycling requires similar layouts and design frameworks as walking. Some of the built and functional elements of each fabric are detailed in Figure 9.2. Of course, there are other ways of classifying

	Active Transport Fabrics	Public Transport Fabrics	Private Car Fabrics
Distance between commonly accessed destinations	Closely congregated 0-2 km	Mixed, some uses closely congregated, others more dispersed 2-20 km	Dispersed 8-20 km
Density	High	High to medium	Low
Diversity of land uses	Heterogeneous	Mostly heterogeneous but some homogenous zones of residential and employment lands	Homogenous
Car parking provision	Low	Low to medium	High
Dominant mode	Walking and cycling	Public transport, walking and cycling	Private car use
Street design	Grid like, easy to navigate	Grid like, easy to navigate, prioritises public transport stops as destinations	Heterogeneous, link roads prioritised, finer grained streets subordinate to the primary road network

Figure 9.2 Characteristics of urban fabrics relevant to transport

Source: Adapted from Newman and Kenworthy 2015

urban areas to understand their inherent transport networks, but we find that the urban fabrics theory works well in an Australian context. This is particularly so because the schema enables respect for the existing fabric, including its car dependence, facilitating moving beyond entirely car-based cities.

In reality, Australian cities and towns have quite complex combinations of all three urban fabrics. Until quite recently, however, stakeholders in transport planning (including government and a sizeable proportion of the general public) have treated each part of the city as though it is either already part of a private car urban fabric or soon will be. A less car-dependent metropolis obviously requires increased consideration of active and public transport urban fabrics. Yet our healthy transport planning aim—to transition away from the harms of private car use while still enabling equitable access—will not be attained by simply replacing, or overlaying, our existing private car urban fabrics with active and public transport urban fabrics. On the contrary, rejuvenation of urban fabrics towards those more supportive of active and public transport can only be successfully achieved in a context of respect for constraints of the existing automobile urban fabric. Further, all of the elements—both the forms and functions—of the desired and existing fabrics must be considered in any rejuvenation or initial development attempt. Failure to provide some, but not all, elements of an active or public transport urban fabric within an automobile urban fabric can result in the new fabrics failing in their function (see Box 9.1).

Box 9.1   The dire consequences of failing to consider all elements of urban fabrics in attempting change

There are plenty of examples from both Australia and around the world of the dire consequences of failing to consider all urban fabrics in any attempt at transition. We present two brief accounts here. The first is from the city of Mumbai, although this story could be applied to any number of developing cities coping with growing urban populations. Mumbai has the dense urban form of a public transport urban fabric; however, the city has yet to build efficient mass public transport services. As a consequence, the city is increasingly saturated with automobiles and motorcycles, with resultant traffic congestion, restricted access and poor health. While Australia's cities will likely never be as dense as Mumbai, we can still learn from these experiences of managing rapid urban population growth. Australia's planners must ensure a serious commitment to the provision of public transport for proposed higher-density developments <u>prior</u> to increasing density and mixing uses.

The second account is of a lower-density development on greenfield land in Melbourne. Selandra Rise, located 52 kilometres southeast of the Melbourne CBD, is a master-planned community covering approximately 12 hectares and containing 1,223 dwellings. Elements of walking and cycling urban fabrics were prioritised in its design, epitomised by grid-like, legible streets, footpath and cycleway provisions and the inclusion of easy-to-access recreational destinations. This development has been studied in depth by Cecily Maller, who has led a team from Victoria's RMIT

University to undertake a longitudinal analysis of the health of Selandra Rise residents. A key conclusion is that although the new development has elements of active transport urban fabrics, its location as an 'island' situated within a wider catchment of private car urban fabric renders this community car-dependent (Nicholls et al. 2017).

From Private Car to Active and Public Transport Urban Fabrics?

Two of the hallmarks of a city reliant on private car use are as follows:

1. Complex road networks accommodating flexible and autonomous ways of travelling
2. Long distances between uses

Any attempt to shift an urban area towards less private car use, while retaining equity of access, must aim to do the following:

1. Accommodate the levels of complexity, autonomy and flexibility characteristic of life in Australian urban areas
2. Remove the need to travel long distances by bringing the things we need and want to access closer together

Presented below are some of the ways these aims can be accomplished.

Accommodating Flexibility and Autonomy

Because cars provide freedom from the timetables and fixed routes of public transport, they enable flexibility and a sense of autonomy to where and when people travel. In Australian urban areas, this freedom results in abundant networks of local and arterial roads and freeways aimed at accommodating (and indeed encouraging) large traffic flows. In the way Australians generally live and travel, the flexibility of the car is translated into lives made up of complex and multiple journeys. Many of us invest emotion and energy in rushing to perform multiple activities sequentially across various distances. Think of a working parent driving first to childcare, then to work, managing a stop at the gym and a quick trip to the supermarket before rushing across the city in time to drop a second child to evening netball practice. We expect to travel spontaneously and erratically, responding just in time to changed plans and places, accommodating the demands of flexible activities, friends and family. As time has passed and Australian cities have become defined by automobile urban fabrics, our complex road networks, long distances between uses and appreciation of autonomous travel have sapped the funds, land and political will away from investment in alternative transport types. As described in the cycle of automobility (Figure 9.1), this has further enshrined the dominance of the private car as the only option for access, regardless of the fact that many people would actually like to use the car less.

In seeking to moderate the health impacts of the private car by encouraging the use of other modes, we need to enable new and existing active and public transport urban fabrics to compete with the flexibility and autonomy enabled by our cars. In addition to removing the need to travel long distances by mixing uses and increasing densities (discussed below), there are many ways that alternative transport modes can achieve flexibility and autonomy. The first is to provide a public transport network that, supplemented with walking and cycling, can be used as the major transport system in the city. This may seem obvious, but in most, if not all, Australian cities, public and active transport networks only fulfil a very limited array of trips, such as the journey to work from the suburbs to a central CBD (Kent and Mulley 2017).

For shorter distances—such as in inner urban areas where density is already high—light rail (tram) systems are a viable option. These are slower systems with more stops, making it more likely that the people who live and work around these networks are within a walkable distance of an access point. For longer distances—such as those bridging the lower densities of suburban areas or connecting these areas to centres—heavy rail (train) networks, supplemented with buses to provide access, are more feasible. Both types of networks form corridors between denser sub-centres, which are built around active transport urban fabrics that contain all the beneficial qualities of a higher-density, walkable precinct. In addition to providing the network and ensuring it is accessible from the places where people live, work and visit, the system needs to be optimised to ensure a high quality of service. In the context of echoing the flexibility and autonomy of the private car, this means serious attention to detail. In short, we want Australia's public transport infrastructure to be all of the things that make private car use appealing: easy to use, predictable, flexible, comfortable and, ultimately, adaptable to the complex tasks and timetables that make up our modern lives. The basics of these details are presented in Box 9.2. For readers interested in further detail from the Australian context, we recommend consulting the informative website of the Public Transport Research Group based at Monash University, Victoria: http://publictransport researchgroup.info/projects/.

Box 9.2   Enhancing the appeal of public transport in car-dependent cities

To be appealing, public transport needs to emulate the convenience of the private car. There are many ways to do this, and with growing access to technology, these measures are increasingly innovative. Some suggestions to make public transport easy and pleasant to use are as follows:

- Provide real-time passenger information using reliable mobile apps and electronic screens at bus stops and stations to enhance the usability and predictability of the system
- Standardise ticketing to facilitate swift and easy transfer between modes
- Provide comfortable, safe and clean stations, shelters and transport interiors
- In both waiting areas and on public transport itself, provide places to sit and store goods such as groceries
- Provide climate control—air-conditioning in summer and heating in winter
- Provide 'time-out' spaces on transport, such as quiet carriages, where loud conversations and mobile phone use are discouraged
- Ensure that the system is universally physically accessible to all users, including parents with young children, the frail elderly and others with limited mobility or vision impairment
- Ensure that timetables and infrastructure accommodate different types of trips, such as those that need to be taken on the weekends, late at night or early in the morning and those that require an element of load-carrying.

While public transport systems can strive for flexibility and autonomy, active and public transport urban fabrics will really raise their appeal in Australia when they are coupled with on-demand options that give users temporary access to the freedom of a private car without the personal and environmental costs of ownership. These services, sometimes known as 'paratransit' (because they are in between active, public and private car transport modes), can fill the gaps in timetables, networks and capacity left by active and public transport in Australia's automobile urban fabrics. Services include traditional taxis and other on-demand ride-share options (such as Uber) as well as commercial car sharing, which is gaining popularity in Australia's larger cities (see Box 9.3). Although we do not yet have Australian data to demonstrate the impact of paratransit on vehicle kilometres travelled (VKT) or car ownership rates, there are many international studies revealing that paratransit users travel less by car and are less likely to own a vehicle. By providing access to a car without ownership, these services can make the decision to go car-free more feasible in the parts of our cities where public transport and walkable urban fabrics satisfy most trips but not all.

Box 9.3   Commercial car sharing in Sydney

Commercial car sharing is a for-profit service that provides members with access to a fleet of vehicles on a short-term (typically half-hourly) basis. After becoming a member of a car sharing organisation, the user can book a car online using a dedicated website or smart phone app. The car is then accessed using an electronic key card or key fob, and members are billed at the end of the month for time and/or kilometres travelled. Cars are located in central business districts, residential areas and major employment centres as well as at public transit stations. In Australia, we have mainly round-trip car-sharing, in that the car sharer must return the car to the same place it was accessed. In between bookings, idle car-share cars usually occupy dedicated parking bays (sometimes referred to as 'pods'—'points of departure') positioned on or off the street.

Ninety percent of car sharing in Sydney's metropolitan region is operated by GoGet (Kent and Dowling 2016b). Founded by two individuals, the business began with four cars in 2002 and has expanded quickly. In 2018, GoGet had more than 1,500 cars across Sydney.

Anecdotally, GoGet claims that its membership is primarily drawn from professionals living in the inner city, and that its members travel fewer kilometres and own fewer cars than non-members. Jennifer and Robyn Dowling of the University of Sydney have undertaken research to examine member motivations to be part of a car sharing initiative. They found users were attracted to:

- the convenience car sharing provides in a congested, public transport–challenged city like Sydney, particularly where on-street car parking is at a premium;
- the financial savings derived; and
- an appreciation of the environmental benefits of not owning a car.

Interestingly, the health benefits of living life with less car dependence are not emphasised.

Bringing Uses Closer Together

The second aim of a transport system transitioning away from car use must be to decrease distances that need to be travelled to access the things required for a happy and healthy life. The long distances between uses in automobile urban fabrics have come about because cars can travel faster than walking, cycling and public transport. As a result, in automobile urban fabrics, it does not matter if we live a long way from where we work or the people with whom we like to socialise, because we can easily bridge that distance by car. To promote active and public transport, we need to reduce distances and bring the things and people we need and like to access closer together. In short, this will mean that, for example, our favourite supermarket, hairdresser and maths coach, as well as our work-place or place of study, are more likely to be close to where we would like to live. It also makes it easier and more economically viable to provide a public transport network that links these places. This does not necessarily reduce the number of trips we might make or even the time we spend travelling. It does, however, make walking, cycling and public transport a more viable option for accessing everything we need.

There are two key planning outcomes required to reduce distances between uses in Australian urban areas—and it is no surprise that these are the features of walkable and (usually) public transport urban fabrics—they are:

- increased densities (of residential, commercial and other uses); and
- mixed uses that incorporate regularly accessed destinations such as schools, shops and places of employment.

For the corridors that make up public transport urban fabrics to be economically, physically and socially viable, they need to have sufficient areas of residential and commercial density strung along their stops and stations. These areas of higher density and mixed uses around stops and stations are often referred to as 'transit-oriented development' or TODs. It is these higher-density neighbourhoods that become the walking urban fabrics because in these areas, shops, services and other places of interest or necessity are more varied (through a mixing of uses) and closer. While the densification of Australia's cities has some questionable impacts on health and liveability, higher densities of all land uses across our cities are a key component of any shift away from private car dependency. Of utmost importance, however, is that densification *on its own* will not encourage public and active transport use. The destinations, mixed uses, transport infrastructure and design quality must also be in place, *before* communities move into higher density. We discuss density and health in more detail in the introduction to Part III—Domains of the Built Environment.

Once distances are reduced so that walking, cycling and public transport become more viable options, planners must concentrate on the design elements that make these modes of transport enjoyable, safe and obvious options. The specific design characteristics of a walking/cycling urban fabric are well researched, and we cannot hope to cover this body of work in a comprehensive way here. We provide more detail on guidelines for walking and cycling, including a comprehensive discussion of distance, density, diversity, destinations and design (also known as the D principles for active transport), in Chapter 3—Planning for Physical Activity. We also refer you to the list of design features for public transport facilities and operations in Box 3.2 as well as the resources in Appendix Two. In short, these are the finishing touches of places where shorter distances already support walking and cycling for transport as well as public transport use. They are the footpath and cycleway treatments that make walking and cycling safe and easy. They include the strategic provision of shade, lighting, signage, seating and bike parking. They extend to include the design of the walking and cycling network to ensure that it is well connected to surrounding uses and intuitively laid out. While these details are just as important as density, diversity and destinations, they, too, will not necessarily result in increased active transport on their own. The need to travel distances that are not walkable or comfortably undertaken on a bike must be reduced in Australian cities before a large-scale shift to active and public transport is possible.

The Future of Healthy Transport in Australia

This chapter has thus far established that, in Australia, a healthy transport network will require the impacts and use of the private car to be tempered while still enabling access to all the things that contribute to a happy and healthy life. In Australian cities and towns, this generally means integrating active and public transport urban fabrics into existing automobile urban fabrics. This in turn requires attainment of the mutually reinforcing goals of a flexible transport system and a reduction in the distances between uses.

Even if distances are reduced and flexibility provided, Australians are so attached to private car use that our planners will need to work hard to lure people out of the comfort of their cars. We are a car-dependent and, for many, car-loving nation. There is, however, hope yet for a transport transition. A serendipitous combination of congested road networks, technological developments and cultural shifts in preferences is prompting some to suggest that we will soon see decreases in car reliance. These are trends on which Australia's transport planners need to capitalise, with the first step being explicit recognition that even Australians will not endure too much wasted time stuck in traffic!

How Traffic Congestion Could Lead to Healthier Transport

To explain our aversion to traffic congestion, we draw upon a key concept in transport planning, the Marchetti constant (Marchetti 1994). This is a transport planning edict that estimates a universal travel time budget of around 60 minutes on average per person each day. This means that although city structure, transport systems and technologies might change, people gradually adjust their lives to their conditions so that the average travel time per day stays approximately constant at one hour long. Australian transport planners have applied the Marchetti constant to transport practices in 41 cities around the world (Newman and Kenworthy 2011). They found that it generally holds true, even in our digitally networked modern lives.

This finding has important implications for healthy transport planning. If people have a consistent travel time budget, that is, a stable daily amount of time that they make available for travel, investment in infrastructure that saves travel time will not necessarily decrease the amount we travel. Instead, it appears people simply reinvest travel time saved in travelling a longer distance. While this is not particularly an issue if people are travelling by healthier modes (particularly walking and cycling), it does call into question the idea of building more roads to reduce the amount of time spent in cars. This is a concept known as latent demand, or induced traffic growth, and it is one of the key arguments used (and often ignored) against new road and motorway projects in Australia.

In the simplest terms, latent demand is demand that exists but, for any number of reasons, is suppressed by the inability of the road network to handle it—usually indicated by a congested road system. It is the travel people would like to do but might avoid because the travel time cost is too great due to traffic congestion. Once additional capacity is added to the road network (for example, by building new roads or widening existing ones), the demand that had been latent materialises as actual usage. Research indicates that this generated traffic often fills a significant portion of any capacity added to a congested urban road. This phenomenon has been explored in depth in an Australian context by Michelle Zeibots of the University of Technology Sydney. Her landmark analysis of the concept of derived demand in Australian freeway projects includes an intriguing and robust analysis of the impact of adding extra capacity to Sydney's iconic Harbour Bridge through construction of a tunnel (see Mewton 2005; Zeibots 2007). The tunnel project was completed in 1992, and the analysis suggests it resulted in a substantial shift away from public modes to car use purely because the option was there.

In reality, as much as it is a derided fact of life in many Australian cities, congestion on our roads is a very effective way to support public and active transport modes. Tackling traffic congestion through the provision of yet more roads, which subsequently become congested, misses an opportunity to bring road speeds down, increasing the appeal of public transport. In fact, because the realities of road construction have fallen short of demand, this is already occurring in our cities. In 1970, the ratio of metropolitan and suburban rail speeds to road speeds was 0.89:1.0, meaning the average speed of our trains was 32% slower than that experienced on Australian roads. By 2005, this ratio had tipped to 1.08:1.0, meaning rail speeds are now actually (slightly) faster than car travel (Newman et al. 2013). This is a global phenomenon. It is one of the founding facts underpinning the theory of peak car—a very slow but discernible decrease in private car dominance (Goodwin 2012). Perhaps the limits of global car use have been reached, with growth now stabilising and, to a degree, even contracting.

Declining Cultural Appreciations of Car Use

In addition to structural limits on private car use imposed by congestion and lack of space for 'yet more' road building in Australian cities, there is some evidence emerging that the nation's cultural appreciation of private, car-based travel is receding. Together with colleagues at Monash University, Alexa Delbosc has pioneered investigations into the transport practices of the millennial generation (those born between 1983 and 2000). Using data on driver licensing in Australia, this team has identified some of the reasons young people in Australia are embracing alternative modes, delaying licensure or at least seeking other avenues to experience freedom and demonstrate maturity. They have found that millennials prefer living in inner urban areas and are happy to use a combination of transport modes to satisfy their travel needs. Indeed, according to this research, very few millennials showed a strong preference for cars. However, the research does suggest that as millennials approach adult milestones, such as having children, the difficulty in finding suitable housing near public transport may push some into neighbourhoods where car use is the only practical option (Delbosc and Nakanishi 2017).

A degree of the desired taming of the private car is therefore emerging already. It seems that our cities and people may be reaching the limit to which they will support automobile urban fabrics, with road congestion slowly shrinking the amount of distance we get for our travel time budget. Improved public and active transport infrastructure and decreased distances between uses are making the choice of active and public transport modes an easier and more logical one, and Australia's planners must take advantage of these developments.

Is Australian Transport Policy Lagging Behind Public Preferences?

At the beginning of this chapter, we introduced the 'system of automobility' (Figure 9.1). At the time of writing, many Australians are questioning the place of the private car in our culture and cities. However, the car's systemic dominance of transport in Australia means that private car use remains embedded deeply in the way our cities are structured and our political economy is played out. A subset of transport research in Australia has explored the way policy-making continues to prioritise the private car in decision-making. Transport policy experts Carey Curtis and Nicholas Low have examined transport planning practices around the country to reveal a dominant and deep-seated 'path-dependent' culture of road construction in Australian cities (Curtis and Low 2012). Path dependence means the continuation of an undesirable course of action—in this case an overt emphasis on planning for private car use—despite the presence of rational reasons to do otherwise. This rationalisation in Australia comes from cultural shifts towards support for better accessibility and public transport provision and acknowledgement of the infrastructural limits of congestion, both outlined above. This work has been complemented by the work of one of Australia's leading transport researchers, Crystal Legacy, which proves that we continue to invest in private car urban fabrics either instead of or, at best, parallel to investments in walking and public transport urban fabrics (Legacy et al. 2017).

Interrupting the path dependence of private car urban fabrics—and breaking the cycle of automobility—requires more than simple behaviour change. It needs a full-scale reorientation of the policy and governance structures that affect the way our cities are configured. Perhaps more so than our other 'Domains of the Built Environment', transport planning and land use planning have traditionally been practised in Australia as parallel, rather than integrated, functions. For example, in New South Wales, the transport and urban planning roles of State government are divided into two separate portfolios, each maintaining its own processes and timeframes of strategic planning, statutory regulation and infrastructural provision. Functions are similarly divided vertically between levels of government, with separate jurisdictions responsible for different infrastructures. Further complicating matters has been the piecemeal inclusion of Federal government funding initiatives, which, since 2013, have focused exclusively on the funding of major road projects. Ideally, healthier transport networks in Australia will require more effective integration of land use and transport planning policy both vertically between levels of governance and horizontally between government agencies. More radically, this could entail dissolution of the false dichotomy between land use and transport agencies altogether. To capture the rising tide of cultural appreciations of walking and public transport urban fabrics, this integration also needs to prioritise community consultation, participation and education.

Conclusion

The link between transport and health can seem obvious. Since the 1970s, for example, Australia, like most developed nations, has pursued an aggressive and successful road safety agenda to prevent the devastating effects of road injuries and deaths. In the early 1980s, recognition of the respiratory impacts of vehicle emissions provoked a fast-paced nationwide embrace of regulations to install catalytic converters in all Australian cars. There are, however, more subtle links between modes of accessibility and our health. These include the way that transport regulates the time and energy we have available for self-care and extends to determining the way we care for and interact with others. In short, a defective transport system can quickly undermine many of the other aspects of healthy built environments.

This chapter has outlined a way forward for a healthy transport system in Australia. Such a system must be based on one key goal: to transition away from the harms of private car use while still enabling equitable access. The following chapter outlines a series of different uses people need to access and ways health can be placed at the forefront of their design and distribution.

References

Banister, D. (2011) Cities, mobility and climate change. *Journal of Transport Geography*, 19(6) pp. 1538–1546.

Bureau of Infrastructure, Transport and Regional Economics (2015) *Traffic and Congestion Cost Trends for Australian Capital Cities*, Information Sheet 74, Department of Infrastructure and Regional Development, Canberra.

Bureau of Infrastructure, Transport and Regional Economics (2017) *Road trauma Australia 2016 Statistical Summary*, Department of Infrastructure and Regional Development, Canberra.

Centre for Accident Research and Road Safety Queensland (CARRS-Q) (2012) *State of the Road: A Fact Sheet of the Centre for Accident Research and Road Safety–Queensland*, CARRRS-Q, Queensland University of Technology, Kelvin Grove, QLD.

Climate Council (2017) *Fact Sheet: Transport Emissions: Driving Down Car Pollution in Cities*, Climate Council, Sydney, NSW.

Curtis, C. and Low, N. (2012) *Institutional Barriers to Sustainable Transport*, Ashgate, Aldershot.

Delbosc, A. and Nakanishi, H. (2017) A life course perspective on the travel of Australian millennials. *Transportation Research Part A: Policy and Practice*, 104 pp. 319–336.

Goodwin, P. (2012) Three views on 'Peak car'. *World Transport Policy and Practice*, 17(4) pp. 8–17.

Hickman, R., Ashiru, O. and Banister, D. (2010) Transport and climate change: Simulating the options for carbon reduction in London. *Transport Policy*, 17(2) pp. 110–125.

Jacobs, J. (1961) *The Death and Life of Great American Cities–The Failure of Town Planning*. Penguin Books, Middlesex.

Kaufmann, V., Bergman, M. M. and Joye, D. (2004) Motility: Mobility as capital. *International Journal of Urban and Regional Research*, 28(4) pp. 745–756.

Kent, J. L. (2014a) Carsharing as active transport: What are the potential health benefits? *Journal of Transport and Health*, 1(1) pp. 54–62.

Kent, J. L. (2014b) Driving to save time or saving time to drive? The enduring appeal of the private car. *Transportation Research Part A: Policy and Practice*, 65 pp. 103–115.

Kent, J. L. (2014c) Still feeling the car–the role of comfort in sustaining private car use. *Mobilities*, 10(5) pp. 726–747.

Kent, J. L. and Dowling, R. (2016a) The future of Paratransit and DRT: Introducing cars on demand: *Paratransit*, in Mulley, C. and Nelson, J. D. eds., *Paratransit: Shaping the Flexible Transport Future*, Emerald, London.

Kent, J. L. and Dowling, R. (2016b) "Over 1000 Cars and No Garage": How Urban Planning Supports Car (Park) Sharing. *Urban Policy and Research* pp. 1–13.

Kent, J. L. and Mulley, C. (2017) Riding with dogs in cars: What can it teach us about transport practices and policy? *Transportation Research Part A: Policy and Practice*, 106 pp. 278–287.

Kjellstrom, T. E., Neller, A. and Simpson, R. W. (2002) Air pollution and its health impacts: The changing panorama. *Medical Journal of Australia*, 177(11) pp. 604–608.

Legacy, C., Curtis, C. and Scheurer, J. (2017) Planning transport infrastructure: Examining the politics of transport planning in Melbourne, Sydney and Perth. *Urban Policy and Research*, 35(1) pp. 44–60.

Marchetti, C. (1994) Anthropological invariants in travel behavior. *Technological Forecasting and Social Change*, 47(1) pp. 75–88.

Mewton, R. (2005) Induced traffic from the Sydney Harbour tunnel and gore hill freeway. *Road and Transport Research*, 14(3) pp. 24–33.

Miller, D. ed. (2001) *Car Cultures*, Berg Publishers, Oxford.

Milner, A., Badland, H., Kavanagh, A. and Lamontagne, A. D. (2017) Time spent commuting to work and mental health: Evidence from 13 waves of an Australian cohort study. *American Journal of Epidemiology*, 186(6) pp. 659–667.

Newman, P. and Kenworthy, J. (2011) 'Peak car use': Understanding the demise of automobile dependence. *World Transport Policy and Practice*, 17(2) pp. 31–42.

Newman, P. and Kenworthy, J. (2015) *The End of Automobile Dependence: How Cities Are Moving Beyond Car-Based Planning*, Island Press, Washington, DC.

Newman, P., Kenworthy, J. and Glazebrook, G. (2013) Peak car use and the rise of global rail: Why this is happening and what it means for large and small cities. *Journal of Transportation Technologies*, 3(4) pp. 272–287.

Nguyen, D. (2010) Evidence of the impacts of urban sprawl on social capital. *Environment and Planning B: Planning and Design*, 37(4) pp. 610–627.

Nicholls, L., Phelan, K. and Maller, C. (2017) 'A fantasy to get employment around the area': Long commutes and resident health in an outer Urban master-planned estate. *Urban Policy and Research*, 36(1) pp. 48–62.

Robinson, D. L. (2005) Air pollution in Australia: Review of costs, sources and potential solutions. *Health Promotion Journal of Australia*, 16(3) pp. 213–220.

Victoria Transport Policy Institute (2018) *Online Transportation Demand Management Encyclopedia*, www.vtpi.org/tdm [Accessed 13 August 2018].

World Health Organization (2000) *Transport, Environment and Health*, World Health Organization, Geneva.

Zeibots, M. (2007) *Before and After the Motorway, Part 1: A Review of Methodologies Used to Investigate the Occurrence of Induced Traffic Growth in International and Australian Cities*, Institute for Sustainable Futures, University of Technology Sydney, Sydney, NSW.

10 Commercial, Service and Employment Spaces

Introduction

This is the final chapter in Part III, Domains of the Built Environment. We have already explored many of the major uses in Australia's urban areas—homes, public spaces and the transport networks that provide connectivity. Now we turn to considering some of the other spaces and places that make up urban Australia. We concentrate on three types of uses integral to a healthy built environment: employment spaces, health-care spaces and school spaces.

Healthy Planning: Australia's Spaces of Employment

The way planning interacts with Australia's economic functioning has many health implications, particularly for the equitable distribution of the resources required to live a happy and healthy life. We know that gainful employment is a key determinant of human health. However, the links between work and health are more complex than simply whether or not one has a job. Here, we focus on two specific aspects: the way planning influences access to employment, including how we travel to work, and the way planning can shape healthier workspaces.

Health and Access to Employment

At the beginning of the 21st Century, when the internet became accessible to most, Australia's planners joined their global counterparts in contemplating the idea that increased online connectivity might disperse the spatial and temporal aspects of the way people work. It was thought that emergent technologies of communication could solve the problems associated with burgeoning city populations. Commuting to and from work would be a thing of the past (Alizadeh and Sipe 2013). It is true that the internet allows people to work from 'virtually' anywhere and enables businesses to achieve connectivity without physical proximity. However, a complete disruption of where and when we work has not come to pass.

Although more people are working less regular hours—sometimes in different places (such as at home)—economic activity in Australia remains largely dependent on face-to-face interaction (Blount 2014). This confirms a long-held planning wisdom that people need contact with others to flourish. Indeed, in Australia, we have actually seen steady increases in the number of jobs concentrated in our capital cities, particularly in the central business districts and specialist business parks of those cities. This is associated with a shift from a manufacturing economy to a service/knowledge-based economy focused on industries where innovation and creativity are central to competitive advantage (see Chapter 1—Australia and Australia's Planning). For a complex array of cultural, logistic and political reasons, these industries need to locate in dense urban environments despite the high price premiums attached to these sites. Urban planning in Australian cities has both supported and reacted to this requirement (see Box 10.1). Most notably, although attempts have been made to suburbanise public transport networks, planning has continued to prioritise central business districts as transport hubs. Planners have also supported and enabled residential densification within walking distance of central business districts. Both of these strategic directions have reinforced the concentration of employment opportunities in our inner cities (see Box 10.1).

Box 10.1   Urban planning and the way people work

Urban planning in Australia is not detached from the various structures and processes that shape the way Australians work. For example, the way our urban areas are planned and managed can impact upon workplace safety and access to employment opportunities. There are more complex links between planning and employment, however, including the increasing concerns about the precariousness of employment in Australia (Cassells et al. 2018).

Job security has a complex link to our health and wellbeing. While unemployment in Australia is relatively low (5.5% at the time of writing), we cannot ignore the fact that a permanent, full-time job is increasingly rare. This casualisation of the workforce will have ongoing impacts on Australia's mental and physical health. For example, as elsewhere, the 'gig economy' has recently emerged in Australia. This is a way of working based on people having temporary jobs or doing one-off pieces of work that are paid separately. Workers in the gig economy do not have a sole employer, but instead might work for several organisations. The odd-jobs broker Airtasker, lift-sharing company Uber and food delivery agencies Foodora and Deliveroo are examples of employers popular in Australia. Like other countries, the numbers working in the gig economy in Australia are significant and rising. In 2017, 4.1 million Australians, or 32% of the workforce, had freelanced during 2014 and 2015 (Knox 2017). While still covered by some regulations in all Australian States, these workers are not well protected by Federal Fair Work legislation, with simple things such as working hours and the provision of a safe work environment deemed to be the responsibility of the individual worker rather than the employer. At the heart of these new, less predictable and reliable ways of working is a faster-paced, more competitive and less equitable society. Unequal access to safe and consistent employment paves the way for the deepening divide in Australia between those who have stable jobs and homes and those who do not. The impact of this divide and the role of urban planning in its perpetuation are further addressed in Chapter 11—Reflections on Principles of Healthy Planning.

Accordingly, planning has helped to shape and respond to the ongoing concentration of Australia's economic activity in the nation's cities. It is this concentration, above all else, that makes Australia such an urban nation, with most people either choosing or needing to live in capital cities to access employment. Job location is frequently a key determinant of residential location and, of course, a defining aspect of how we travel to and from work. If employment is not located close to sufficient housing for workers, or if it is situated in places where housing is unaffordable, people are either forced into long commutes or are unable to find the job for which they have trained—or even find any job at all.

In part reflecting the issue of housing affordability and the centralisation of jobs in cities, Australia has some of the longest average commute times in the world. Research conducted in 2017 shows that Australians spent an average of 80 minutes per day commuting, 20 minutes longer than in Germany and almost double the average commute times in Japan (Holmes 2017). However, averages can be misleading. Sydney's average commute of just over 60 minutes pales in significance compared with the journeys of those who spend over five hours every day in transit. These 'super commutes' are an increasingly common fact of life for people pushed out of our jobs-rich inner urban areas by high housing prices and inappropriate accommodation options. For these people, stress comes from the opportunity costs of spending such a huge amount of time travelling every day. David Bissel of the University of Melbourne has studied the impacts of long commutes in Australian cities using ethnographic research techniques (Bissel 2015). In this work, participants described the 'parallel lives' they live with their family, children and friends, lamenting the time lost to commuting that could otherwise be spent with family and in the community.

The impact of commutes on health needs to be seen in the context of the fact that many people do prefer to have some kind of a separation—both in time and space—between the place where they work and the place where they live. Research has demonstrated that this is somewhere between 15 and 30 minutes, meaning people are usually relatively happy to travel about 30–60 minutes per day for their journey to and from work (Ory et al. 2004). This confirms the theory of the Marchetti constant described in Chapter 9—Transport, Access and Health. Paring back from the outliers of super commutes mentioned above, the fact remains that almost a quarter of Australians have a commute of 90 minutes or more per day. This stretches the preference implied by the Marchetti constant, and the increasing prevalence of these longer-than-preferred travel times does impact people's health. As an example, research conducted by the Australian Bureau of Transport and Regional Economics combined travel data from Australian capital cities with health data from the longitudinal Household, Income and Labour Dynamics in Australia Survey (HILDA) to reveal that long commutes are associated with a poor sense of wellbeing (Bureau of Infrastructure, Transport and Regional Economics 2016). Australians with longer commutes display lower overall life satisfaction, reduced overall job satisfaction and diminished satisfaction with the amount of free time they have (see Box 10.2).

Box 10.2   Housing key workers

Access to employment is a key component of housing affordability. Urban planner Nicole Gurran and her team from the University of Sydney have recently explored the spatial mismatch between the location of affordable housing and the location of employment opportunities. This Sydney-based research on 'key workers' (such as teachers, police and ambulance and other emergency workers) demonstrates that unaffordable housing is creating a growing divide between where key workers live and work. Although their jobs are spread throughout the metropolitan region, in 2017, a majority of Sydney's 156,000 teachers, nurses, police, firefighters and ambulance and emergency workers lived in the less expensive outer ring areas. Furthermore, the study showed that this trend is intensifying.

Over the decade 2006–2016, inner and middle ring suburbs of Sydney lost up to 21.4% of their key worker populations. The largest influxes of key workers were to the Illawarra (a net gain of 10.5%), Hunter Valley (13.6%) and Southern Highlands (17%)—all areas over 100 kilometres from the Sydney central business district (Gurran et al. 2018).

Health and the Spaces of Working

Our second focus for the link between health and spaces of employment is the way planning affects the actual design of the workplace. Traditionally, healthy workspaces have been conceptualised within the realm of occupational health and safety. Like many other nations, the regulatory framework of occupational health and safety in Australia has a long history. This dates back to the late 19th Century, when regulations were developed to protect factory workers experiencing the most hazardous elements of the Industrial Revolution. Australia imported its initial occupational health and safety regulatory approach from Britain. Today, it is a State, rather than Federal, responsibility. As such, each State has its own legislation and codes of practice, enforced by a State-specific regulatory body. In addition, some States also have special regulations for different industries, particularly mining. While the States have autonomy in their regulation of occupational health and safety, since the 1970s, they have been guided by a national body now known as Safe Work Australia.

The way urban planning intersects with occupational health and safety in Australia is less direct than in many other jurisdictions around the world. In part, this is because our occupational health and safety policies cover both the spaces of work and the way people work—such as hours and procedures. In regard to the latter, urban planning in Australia has little direct influence, although there are some exceptions (see Box 10.2). In the allocation of land for and the design of working spaces, however, planning can intervene. For example, good urban planning can ensure that plots of land are of a sufficient size to accommodate a particular industrial activity safely or use zoning to prohibit the co-location of incompatible functions. In terms of design, the specific guidelines for the basics of a healthy workplace are covered in various building codes, such as the National Construction Code. As with residential buildings, these codes are referenced and enforced by urban planners in the assessment and issuance of development consents and compliance certificates once a building is constructed.

In recent years, there has been considerable focus on the design of healthy office spaces, prompted in part by the emergence of the term 'sick building syndrome' (see, for example, Standing Committee on Public

Works 2001). Research has shown that headaches, respiratory problems, eye strain and fatigue among office workers are directly related to poor ventilation and hours spent in front of computer screens and on phone headsets (Allen et al. 2016). Yet ensuring that office buildings are 'healthy' is a difficult task. In Australian offices, basic features such as ventilation and insulation are regulated by building codes, as mentioned above. But other design features that are known to have a big impact on human health are still not mandated. For example, there is evidence that direct contact with natural elements, including exposure to natural light, can have positive effects on employee productivity and welfare at work—yet there is no legislative requirement for these features to be integrated into new workplace environments or retrofitted into existing places of work.

Nevertheless, mindful of the costs of lost productivity through sick days and reduced capacity, some organisations are investing in the design of healthy office spaces. Air filtered by green walls and other plants is now a reality in many Australian offices, as are sleep pods, lounge areas, games facilities and sensory rooms. By creating well-designed, centrally located eating areas that are fitted with the equipment and ingredients for healthy food preparation, organisations are encouraging employees to make better food choices. Recognising the health risks associated with prolonged periods of sitting (described in Chapter 4—Planning for Physical Activity), employees are increasingly provided with 'sit-stand' desks that can be adjusted to enable both sitting and standing while working. Finally, some organisations realise that the simple provision of contact with natural environments, including natural ventilation, views of nature and greenery in the workplace, can improve employees' wellbeing and productivity. For some (lucky) employees, this extends to the ability of people to bring companion animals into the workplace. We discussed the links between health and companion animal ownership in Australia in Chapter 5—Planning for Social Interaction. As a country with one of the highest dog ownership rates in the world, it is not surprising that we are enthusiastic participants in the international 'Take Your Dog to Work' day. Started in the United States in 1990, in Australia, this initiative is promoted each June by the Royal Society for the Protection of Animals (RSPCA), Australia's leading independent, non-government, community-based charity providing animal care and protection services.

We are conscious that the state-of-the art office fitouts described above are generally provided in the name of worker productivity, rather than an intrinsic concern for human health. Using office planning and design to increase productivity can also have negative health effects. While green walls, lounge areas and fully stocked kitchens are now commonplace in many newer Australian offices, so is the concept of activity-based working—another initiative used to enhance productivity for less capital investment in office space. This way of working uses the concept of hot-desking, where employees do not have an assigned workspace. This practice reduces the amount of actual space required to accommodate office workers and is therefore a less expensive option for management than providing each employee with a dedicated desk. In the central business districts of Australia's largest cities, where office space is particularly expensive, this is increasingly commonplace. But research suggests that frequent desk relocations can waste time, and the background noise associated with open-plan working can increase distractions, fatigue and stress (Morrison and Macky 2017). Another criticism of hot-desking is that it denies employees an opportunity to express their identity at work. This in turn can decrease job satisfaction, sense of belonging and general wellbeing. The potential outcome of the consequences of activity-based working, including hot-desking, is a negative impact on mental wellbeing.

A final reflection on the healthy workplace initiatives discussed above is that they only benefit the very few who work in recently constructed or renovated office spaces, where the employer has had the budget to invest in workplace wellbeing. These privileges can generally be found in the offices of successful corporations whose employees are already relatively well paid. For every Australian that works in a traditional desk job, approximately five are employed in other environments (Australian Bureau of Statistics [ABS] 2018). Most Australians travel to work each day to, for example, a healthcare facility, construction site, school, mine or factory, rather than an air-conditioned office space. In promoting healthy working spaces, it is important to consider the diverse array of both workplaces and the practices people call 'work'.

Healthy Planning: Australia's Hospitals and Primary Healthcare Services

While our entire book is dedicated to the links between health and urban planning, this section has a specific focus on the way urban planning influences the location and design of actual hospitals and healthcare services. Ensuring people have easy and equitable access to such facilities both in times of need and when seeking preventative treatment is an important urban planning concern. Healthcare facilities are also one of the major employers in Australia. Their location and design are important shapers of the wider urban environment and the ability of this environment to promote health and wellbeing. Finally, the place that is a hospital often provides the backdrop for key moments in people's lives. They are the places where we heal, care for others, welcome life and say goodbye. A hospital's design is not simply a matter of making a space that is functional; it is also an opportunity to bring solace and distraction at times when we are at our most vulnerable.

Hospital and Health Service Distribution

The distribution of hospitals and health services is the responsibility of the health department in each Australian State. Every department has its own infrastructure section that works with other government agencies, such as transport and urban planning, to determine where facilities are required. Indeed, for many years, this was the primary way urban planners interacted with health professionals—approving and advising on the appropriate location for health facilities. This was until the (re)emergence of the more holistic relationship between health and planning described in this book.

Each State's large and influential government health portfolio has had the unenviable task of providing health services to an increasingly diverse, expanding and decentralised community. Our oldest hospitals are located in central areas and are now often connected to larger health and education precincts that have flourished to become major hubs for employment, investment, infrastructure provision and, increasingly, residential density. The Prince of Wales/University of NSW health education precinct is an example of a hospital anchored to a major university now attracting public transport infrastructure investment (Bunker et al. 2018).

The period between 1955 and 1975 brought a major escalation in hospital construction, with most new services located in suburban and regional areas designed to be closer to their catchment populations. Since this time, and particularly within Australia's larger cities, there has been a distinct reversion to policies that favour consolidating and extending existing hospitals, rather than constructing hospitals in new areas. This results in fewer, but larger, hospitals. While such an approach has undeniable benefits from the perspective of managing health service delivery (for example, providing economies of scale to reduce operational costs and concentrate teaching and research activities), the urban planning implications are less positive. Of particular concern is that this approach renders transport to and from hospitals much more difficult for the general population. Hospitals are the places where people experience some of the most stressful moments in life. The trauma of attending and visiting hospital in Australian cities is often accompanied by the added tension of a complex cross-city trip to an unfamiliar neighbourhood where parking is often scarce and expensive. Another concern with the consolidation approach is that as employment and study hubs, swathes of workers and students travel to and from large hospital precincts each day. These movements are often at unpredictable times of day or night, making the provision of public and active transport networks to these areas particularly complex. Encouraging healthcare workers to use alternatives to the comfort and convenience of the private car is further complicated by long shifts and immensely physical and stressful working practices. A final concern with hospital consolidations is that these precincts are less likely to contain an adequate amount of affordable housing for the key workers and students.

The government response to these issues in Australia has first been to invest in day surgery so that patients can be discharged within 24 hours. The result is less time in hospital and reduced stress on carers because the need to travel to the hospital precinct is reduced. Second has been investment in ambulatory care services that do not require hospital admission and instead strengthen the role of the general practitioner. This means that coordinated care can be delivered through clinics located in the community. Third has been prioritisation of 'ageing in place' and provision of other in-home services. Finally, electronic medical records that connect patient care across the life course have allowed many hospitals to define their boundaries electronically, rather than spatially. This also facilitates hospital-style care outside the institutional setting, further satisfying the need for localised services and minimising the need to travel.

Hospital Design in Australia

In addition to influencing the distribution of hospital and health services, urban planners in Australia also determine, in part, the way they are designed. The basic details of hospital design are contained in the Australasian Health Facility Guidelines, which are maintained by the Australasian Health Infrastructure Alliance. The Alliance is a public sector collaboration to promote better planning, procurement and management of health capital assets. It has custodianship of the Australasian Health Facility Guidelines which are applied by urban planners, engineers and building compliance officers to assess applications for health facilities.

Hospital design in Australia has a somewhat chequered history, in that it has enjoyed times of great innovation and endured periods now recognised as less remarkable. The first hospital of the type envisioned in the European paradigm was not constructed in Australia until over 25 years after European settlement. This was the Sydney Hospital—an amalgam of three Georgian-style buildings opened in 1816. This initial attempt at hospital design in Australia was met with contempt, immediately prompting an adverse report from the then Government Architect, Sir Francis Greenway. During the early 20th Century, however, Australia enjoyed a special status as one of the world's most progressive countries for hospital design. Architects such as Sir Arthur Stephenson and Leighton Irwin introduced many innovative concepts into design, adapting European concepts to Australia's climate. Natural light and fresh air were central to these designs, as was the ability to accommodate new technologies such as steam sterilisation and radiography (Kerr 2013).

Hospital design during the boom period from 1955 to 1975 was based primarily on functional need, and many of the facilities constructed during this time had a very sparse and institutional feel. The less immediate needs of patients were generally not given priority. Concurrent improvements in technologies of air-conditioning and other mechanical systems enabled emergence of deep-plan, inwardly focused buildings. These structures permitted functional working arrangements between different hospital departments but also ensured patients and healthcare providers were cut off from access to external views and fresh air.

Skip forward to the post-millennium period, and worldwide, the architectural design of healthcare facilities is a discipline in itself and one to which Australia makes a highly visible contribution. In short, there has been a global reorientation towards a holistic and humanistic perspective in the design of hospitals. Evidence-based design, patient-centred design and salutogenic perspectives are combined to once again emphasise natural light, fresh air, natural colours and materials and access to views and green space (Dilani 2008). These are routinely considered to be vital attributes of healing environments. The teams developing hospitals are increasingly multidisciplinary, with architects and designers working alongside specialists in sociology, psychology, the arts and biophysical sustainability to produce hospital environments that promote a holistic view of wellness.

Incorporating Nature Into Australian Hospitals

Epitomising this more holistic orientation is renewed emphasis on the incorporation of nature into healthcare settings. Popularised by Roger Ulrich's seminal study (1984), there is now abundant and robust evidence that simply being exposed to plants, animals and other elements of the natural world can provide patients, visitors and staff at hospitals with a range of health benefits. In recognition of this, hospital facilities are increasingly designed to provide restorative and therapeutic environments.

The notion of restorative environments is underpinned by attention restoration theory (Kaplan and Kaplan 2003). The basic premise of this theory is that natural elements provide multiple objects of fascination, particularly in built-up urban environments. Even the motion of leaves in the wind, birdsong and patterns and shadows on the ground enable restful occupation of the mind of the type required to recover both physically and mentally from the inevitable stress associated with hospital life and recovery from illness. The Royal Children's Hospital Melbourne, which opened in 2012, has been designed explicitly to integrate nature and natural elements. The basis for the design was developed by Ray Green, a landscape architect at the University of Melbourne. Situated in a parkland setting, the aim was to integrate as much as possible with the park to provide patients, staff and visitors with a connection to the external world around them. This was done through an emphasis on views (particularly for patients while lying or seated) and use of materials, colours and even sounds that reference the exterior park. Actual nature (flora and fauna) and water features are common throughout the hospital's interior, as are rooftop gardens, greenhouses, vertical gardens, aquariums, planter boxes and terrariums. Its crowning salute to nature as a healing force is an open-air enclosure that is home to five cheeky meerkats. The enclosure is located in a waiting area, with staff from the Melbourne Zoo arriving to care for the meerkats and provide education sessions each day. The animals provide distraction and a learning experience for children who are both visiting and undergoing treatment. The animals have also become a focus for anxious carers and stressed staff.

Going one step further, many recently constructed hospital and health facilities now provide working gardens specifically for patients to tend. These facilities are a step beyond the simple provision of nature in care settings because they are accompanied by a specific treatment goal. This might be, for example, a focus for mindfulness and meditation or an environment for movement restoration. One such therapeutic environment was built into the Royal Talbot Rehabilitation Centre, also in Melbourne. The Royal Talbot provides rehabilitative treatment to patients recovering from extreme trauma, including acquired brain and spinal cord injuries, upper and lower limb amputation and acquired neurological disorders. Patients are often admitted for long periods of time. The restorative garden space enables engagement in potting plants and tending the garden and provides a space for relaxation and a place to receive visitors.

Hospital and Health Services in Rural Australia

Australia's vast land size has demanded resourcefulness in dealing with the provision of health services in remote and rural areas. The nation's population geography is outlined in Chapter 1—Australia and Australia's Planning. In summary, although almost 90% of Australians live in cities or larger regional centres, the remaining 10% are spread across a land mass that is almost the size of the United States. These communities are often separated by extreme road distances, making early intervention in illness, as well as education on health promotion and disease prevention, very difficult. To manage this burden of geography, Australian States have generally developed a larger number of smaller facilities in outlying towns that are then supported by a regional hospital. These health centres and hospitals are often one of the most important buildings in the town or region, existing as a major employer and providing a social link for the community to wider structures of governance. In very remote areas, these services are also supported by the Royal Flying Doctor Service—one of the largest and oldest aeromedical organisations in the world.

It is key for planners of health facilities in Australia to recognise that rural and regional facilities are not simply smaller, more isolated versions of their city equivalents. Their design needs to respond to the specific context of the communities they serve. This includes cultural context as well as catering for the unique health needs of those living outside of Australia's dominant cities. Using better facility design to accommodate the needs of Australia's Indigenous communities is particularly important. In Australia, Aboriginal and Torres Strait Islander people generally represent a higher proportion of the population in rural and regional areas, and, as discussed in Chapter 2—Australia's Health, this population is grossly over-represented across most indicators of ill health. Case study research has shown that Indigenous Australians commonly have a relative distrust of the European model of healthcare provision (Isaacs et al. 2010). This is a cynicism generated by the oft-forceful superimposition of western ideas over traditional approaches to healing. This has been done in a way that is at best disrespectful and at worst devastatingly detrimental to physical and mental health. As a result, some Aboriginal and Torres Strait Islander people remain wary of hospital buildings and health facilities. While States maintain guidelines for the design of health facilities for Indigenous Australian communities, the planners and architects involved in these projects must still consult with local traditional owners. The designers need to gain a nuanced understanding of the way a particular community views the journey from illness to wellness, or indeed the journey to death, when this occurs (Peters 2013). In a very practical sense, facilities that serve Aboriginal and Torres Strait Islander communities may need to be designed to include external waiting areas, provision for ceremonies at births and deaths or provision for culturally required segregation at certain times between sexes or age groups. The aspiration should be to provide a facility that is welcoming and respectful of culture as well as effective in treating culturally specific health needs.

Finally, it is worth considering that as the concept of telemedicine becomes more sophisticated, rural and remote communities will be increasingly reliant on online expertise, imparted via either a medical specialist or the patient's community general practitioner or a carer. This has the benefit of enabling patients to remain within their community and can also facilitate more timely interventions. It does, however, rely on robust electronic infrastructure, including the networks that support internet access across Australia's extensive land mass. This infrastructure needs to be embedded in the design and future planning of rural and regional health facilities and hospitals.

Healthy Planning: Australia's Schools

Childhood obesity in Australia is a debilitating and costly health issue. At the time of writing, an estimated 25% of children aged five to 18 were overweight or obese, and this figure is increasing (Australian Institute of Health and Welfare [AIHW] 2016). School environments are the places where children spend a large proportion of their time during their most impressionable years. Schools are therefore places with immense potential to foster healthy habits.

There are many ways school planning can influence health. For example, location can determine whether a child can walk to school. The design of a playground space can shape opportunities for physical activity through formal sports and improvised play. School grounds are also often the spaces where children learn to interact—both with nature and each other. Nevertheless, the way we access and use school grounds becomes irrelevant if we do not allocate adequate space in our urban environments for schools. We therefore start this section by providing an insight into the way schools are distributed across Australia's urban areas.

Schools and School Planning in Australia

Free and compulsory education for children between the ages of six and 14 was introduced in Australia in 1873, three years ahead of England (Campbell and Proctor 2014). Today, school education is provided free for all students in 'public', or 'State', schools, and there are also 'private' schools that charge higher fees.

Although the exact ages of compulsory school attendance vary from State to State, children must generally attend school from the ages of five to 15, with almost 80% of Australian adolescents staying to finish school at approximately age 18 (ABS 2016). This means that most children are at school for 13 years. Most students attend school between around 9.00 am and 3.30 pm, Monday to Friday, and many children are also on school grounds before and after school hours to partake in organised activities such as sports or music. In most States, it is illegal for children, or anyone not authorised, to be on school grounds outside of school hours unless participating in an organised activity. Enforcement of this prohibition is a relatively new phenomenon brought about by workplace health and safety obligations and the common law duty of care that applies to schools (McShane and Wilson 2017). This duty is not time-limited, and so the school could be liable for accidents that occur outside of school hours. As will be discussed below, while safety must be paramount, the cordoning off of school grounds from use for improvised play on weekends and after school misses a great opportunity to provide open spaces in communities where open space is increasingly in demand.

The choice of which public school a child will attend is determined by catchment areas, and the way these catchments are defined varies from State to State. In most States, schools can enrol out-of-catchment students only if sufficient capacity—both existing and projected—is available. While access to a high standard of education is considered a basic right in Australia, there are, inevitably, some public schools that are considered better than others. An increased focus on student testing—and publication of school indicators of quality—has ensured that parents and students are more aware of these differences than ever. It is not unusual for real estate advertisements to cite access to a specific highly ranked school as a selling point for property and for parents to choose where they live based on the area's school. This has planning implications by raising the cost of living around highly ranked schools.

Education (like Health and Transport) is another portfolio managed primarily by State government, with each State maintaining a slightly different approach to school planning and design. The one universal reality for all States is that maintaining existing schools and planning for new ones demand intense collaboration between government agencies. Urban planners work within State government education portfolios to coordinate this collaboration, often crossing the portfolio boundaries of Transport, Health, Treasury, Sport and Recreation, Family and Community Services, Housing and Local Government.

Future Challenges for Schools

The key challenge for school planning in Australia is simply providing enough school space. Although the Australian population is ageing, we have also experienced an unexpected baby boom throughout the first decade of the 21st Century. As a result, in many Australian cities, the population of school-aged children is growing faster than the government can provide space. This conundrum is further exacerbated because the population of school-aged children is growing most dramatically in inner urban areas. These are the areas where planners have focused densification strategies, and land prices are at a premium. This makes it particularly difficult to procure new land for school construction.

Given the magnitude of the growth forecast in school-aged children, the business-as-usual approach to school provision is not viable for the future. There needs to be a substantial shift in the way Australian schools are planned. Most States plan to meet increased demand by prioritising redevelopment of existing school sites over and above the building of new establishments. This might include constructing more classrooms on the same site or providing spaces that are adaptable for multiple uses (such as a set of classrooms that can be transformed into a school hall). New schools are still being built, particularly in greenfield locations, but existing schools are generally expected to accommodate more students than in the past. In New South Wales, for example, the average primary school size is set to rise from 640 students in 2016 to 1,000 students by 2031 (Infrastructure New South Wales 2018).

So how will large schools affect the educational experience and health of Australia's children? Research on their impact is not conclusive. Echoing the common theme in this book, context is all-important, and a successful larger school in one area may be less effective in another. Increased student numbers per school have two key healthy planning considerations: school accessibility by active modes and the provision of enough space for health-promoting activities such as free play. We now discuss each in turn.

Active Transport to School

Allowing schools to accommodate larger numbers of students risks expanding a school's geographic catchment zone. From a healthy planning perspective, this is a concern because it may mean that fewer children live within a walkable or safely ridable distance of where they attend school. This erodes an opportunity for physical activity through an active journey to school. It also expands the geographical footprint of the child's activity sphere outside of school, as birthday parties, school team sports and classmate sleep-overs all become more than a walk away from home. This means that the child is dependent on their carer as a chauffeur if they are to participate in these activities.

The idea of the chauffeured child calls up the concept of 'children's independent mobility', which simply refers to a child travelling without adult supervision. This practice has been severely eroded throughout the latter part of the 20th Century. As outlined in Chapter 9—Transport, Access and Health—this is partly because our car-dependent cities make streets potentially dangerous places for young people. Car dependence and the 'cycle of automobility' (see Figure 9.1) result in longer distances between uses than a child could possibly access on foot. Declining children's independent mobility is also related to an increased awareness of danger from strangers. Child abduction and abuse are universal fears, and in Australia, the constant surveillance of children is often associated with notions of good parenting and cultural expectations of care (Dowling 2000).

For many reasons, including the regularity of the trip and the sociability aspect of sharing time walking with family and friends, the journey to school is a perfect opportunity to foster children's independent mobility and promote physical activity and sociability. It is often while undertaking this journey that Australian kids learn the skills of being mobile within their community. Crossing the road safely, obeying traffic signals, walking on the left side of the footpath—these are all things that can be learned by a child through the regular trip to school. Australia has, however, witnessed an extraordinary decline in the number of children using active transport to get to school. In New South Wales, for example, the proportion of children aged five to nine who walked to school declined from 57.7% in 1971 to 25.5% in 2003. In Melbourne, 55.3% of children walked to school in 1970. By 1994, this figure had fallen to 22.2%, with a concurrent increase in children being driven to school from 14.3% to 43.9% (Schoeppe et al. 2016).

The importance of children's active journeys to school is well researched in the Australian context. Carolyn Whitzman of the University of Melbourne has mapped regulatory contexts supportive of Australian children's independent mobility (Whitzman and Pike 2007). This research found that while it is parental attitudes that ultimately determine how a child travels to and from school, there are many policies that can assist in ensuring the feasibility and safety of an active school commute. These include slowing traffic, not only directly around the school but also within the school neighbourhood. Most States, and some Local government authorities, also maintain several educational programs and initiatives to encourage safe active transport to school. Brisbane City Council in Queensland has been particularly effective in encouraging children to walk, ride or use a scooter to get to school. The Brisbane City Council Active School Travel Program has been in operation since 2007 and includes initiatives such as 'Walking Wheeling Wednesday'—a continuous campaign to encourage students to actively travel to school at least one day a week. 'Park and Stride' is another component of the program that encourages students who are driven to school to walk part of the way. Even walking part of the way to school gives children an opportunity to have some physical activity as well as learn vital pedestrian skills. Anecdotal evaluations of the Brisbane City Active School Travel Program suggest ongoing success.

Using School Space for Healthy Activities

It is the school space outside of the classrooms, halls and offices that is of particular interest to healthy planning. Because our climate is mild relative to many other countries, Australian school children are able to play comfortably outdoors throughout the entire year (wearing a mandatory hat for sun protection in primary schools). It is in these spaces that aspects of all four of our domains for wellbeing can be nurtured. Most obviously, these spaces host physical activity ranging from improvised play to organised sport and games. They are the spaces where children learn to interact with their peers and where the ability to form community connection begins. By providing space for kitchen food gardens and other opportunities for interaction with the biophysical environment, they are also spaces that educate children about the importance of a healthy planet and healthy eating.

Each State maintains a set of design guidelines for the outdoor areas in schools. These stipulate things such as the amount of play space required and the ratio of teaching space infrastructure to core facilities such as libraries, school halls and office areas. Schools are also required to ensure that all facilities comply with a suite of Australian Standards for Playground and Equipment Surfacing (Jeavons et al. 2017). Australia's growing school populations are fostering a new wave of innovation in how to provide spaces for play and time out. Our school planners are currently in pursuit of several novel options to ensure that children have access to the facilities required to be healthy and happy at school. This includes the use of rooftops for play in multistorey schools and organising for uses to be shared with other community activities. When this occurs, the school develops a joint or shared-use agreement. These are arrangements between the school (usually at the discretion of the school's Principal) and the community to share facilities. It might mean opening up a hall on the school grounds for an evening drawing class (shared use) or the more complex option where facilities are actually planned, built and managed by both a school and a partner organisation (joint use). In Ellenbrook, Western Australia, for example, the developer of a residential estate negotiated a joint-use agreement between the State government and Local Council. The agreement delivered a secondary school that shares a library, performance arts centre and sports facilities with the Local Council (Western Australian Department of Sport and Recreation 2011).

The Importance of Balance in Schools

A final note on school environments is the need to maintain a balance when encouraging children to eat healthy food and undertake physical activity. With so many mixed messages about what to eat, how to exercise, the 'obesity crisis', celebrity culture and social media, many children are feeling confused about what is 'healthy'. Sadly, a study undertaken by the Australian Childhood Association showed that amongst 12- to 17-year-olds in Australia, 90% of girls and 68% of boys had been on a diet of some kind (Tucci et al. 2007). It is not surprising, therefore, that over 15% of Australians develop an eating disorder such as anorexia nervosa or bulimia nervosa in their lifetime (Butterfly Foundation 2012). The most common time for this to occur is during adolescence and, increasingly, childhood, and schools are generally the key hosts of this life stage. Childhood and adolescence are times when ideas are formed and bodies are changing. An unhealthy relationship with food and physical activity during this critical period is just as debilitating for children and their families as being overweight or obese. At all junctures, the message must be loud and clear that health and wellbeing are the outcomes of healthy eating and physical activity. Foods in schools should not be labelled 'good' or 'bad', and physical activity should never be conceptualised as a way to burn kilojoules. The emphasis should be on fun and enjoyment, and any focus on shape or size or restrictive or intensely rigid eating practices must be avoided through these vulnerable years and beyond.

Conclusion

This chapter covers some of the different spaces where Australians spend a lot of their time. Spaces of employment, healing and education are fundamental to our lives. As a result, they have enormous potential to foster healthy practices. The need to accommodate a growing population and a marked shift away from government intervention in space and service management are two recurring themes in this chapter. Some of the most serious risks associated with these spaces—long commutes, precarious employment, diminishing community-based healthcare and shrinking school grounds—are also associated with these trends. Of course, this reflects two broader themes in Australia: our changing demography and an increasingly market-led approach to governance. These themes pose real risks to the health of Australians, and the final chapter in this book unpicks some of the pathways between equity, diversity, health and urban planning.

References

Alizadeh, T. and Sipe, N. (2013) Impediments to teleworking in live/work communities: Local planning regulations and tax policies. *Urban Policy and Research*, 31(2) pp. 208–224.

Allen, J. G., MacNaughton, P., Satish, U., Santanam, S., Vallarino, J. and Spengler, J. D. (2016) Associations of cognitive function scores with carbon dioxide, ventilation, and volatile organic compound exposures in office workers: A controlled exposure study of green and conventional office environments. *Environmental Health Perspectives*, 124(6) pp. 805–812.

Australian Bureau of Statistics (2016) *Education and work, Australia, May*, Cat. no. 6227.0, Australian Bureau of Statistics, Canberra.

Australian Bureau of Statistics (2018) *Labour Force, Australia, May*, Cat. no. 6202.0, Australian Bureau of Statistics, Canberra.

Australian Institute of Health and Welfare (2016) *Australia's Health 2016*, Australian Institute of Health and Welfare, Canberra.

Bissell, D. (2015) *Understanding the Impacts of Commuting: Research Report for Stakeholders*, Australian National University, Canberra.

Blount, Y. (2014) Telework: Not business as usual, in Haider, A. ed., *Business Technologies in Contemporary Organizations: Adoption, Assimilation, and Institutionalization*, IGI Global, Hershey, PA, pp. 76–95.

Bunker, R., Freestone, R. and Randolph, B. (2018) Sydney: Growth, globalization and governance, in Hamnett, S. and Freestone, R. eds., *Planning Metropolitan Australia*, Routledge, London.

Bureau of Infrastructure, Transport and Regional Economics (2016) *Lengthy Commutes in Australia*, Report 144, Department of Infrastructure and Regional Development, Canberra, ACT.

Butterfly Foundation (2012) *Paying the Price: The Economic and Social Impact of Eating Disorders in Australia*, Butterfly Foundation, Melbourne.

Campbell, C. and Proctor, H. (2014) *A History of Australian Schooling*, Allen & Unwin, Sydney, NSW.

Cassells, R., Duncan, A., Mavisakalyan, A., Phillimore, J., Seymour, R. and Tarverdi, Y. (2018) *Future of Work in Australia: Preparing for Tomorrow's World*, Bankwest Curtin Economics Centre, Perth.

Dilani, A. (2008) Psychosocially supportive design: A salutogenic approach to the design of the physical environment. *Design and Health Scientific Review*, 1(2) pp. 47–55.

Dowling, R. (2000) Cultures of mothering and car use in suburban Sydney: A preliminary investigation. *Geoforum*, 31(3) pp. 345–353.

Gurran, N., Gilbert, C., Zhang, Y. and Phibbs, P. (2018) *Key Worker Housing Affordability in Sydney*, University of Sydney, Sydney, NSW.

Holmes, A. (2017) *The Countries with the Longest and Shortest Commutes*, 31 March, Dalia Research, https://daliaresearch.com/the-countries-with-the-longest-and-shortest-commutes/ [Accessed 12 July 2018].

Infrastructure New South Wales (2018) *State Infrastructure Strategy 2018–2038*. Infrastructure New South Wales, Sydney, NSW.

Isaacs, A. N., Pyett, P., Oakley-Browne, M. A., Gruis, H. and Waples-Crowe, P. (2010) Barriers and facilitators to the utilization of adult mental health services by Australia's Indigenous people: Seeking a way forward. *International Journal of Mental Health Nursing*, 19(2) pp. 75–82.

Jeavons, M., Jeameson, S. and Elliott, S. (2017) Application of standards and regulations, in Little, H., Elliott, S. and Wyver, S. ed., *Outdoor Learning Environments: Spaces for Exploration, Discovery and Risk-Taking in the Early Years*, Allen & Unwin, Sydney, NSW.

Kaplan, S. and Kaplan, R. (2003) Health, supportive environments, and the reasonable person model. *American Journal of Public Health*, 93(9) pp. 1484–1489.

Kerr, W. (2013) A history of growth. Australian healthcare design, in Copeland, K. ed., *Australian Healthcare Design 2005–2015: A Critical Review of the Design and Build of Healthcare Infrastructure in Australia*, International Academy for Design and Healthy, Brisbane.

Knox, D. (2017) A super gig. *Superfunds Magazine*. 427 pp. 25–27.

McShane, I. and Wilson, C. K. (2017) Beyond the school fence: Rethinking Urban schools in the twenty-first century. *Urban Policy and Research*, 35(4) pp. 472–485.

Morrison, R. L. and Macky, K. A. (2017) The demands and resources arising from shared office spaces. *Applied Ergonomics*, 60 pp. 103–115.

Ory, D. T., Mokhtarian, P. L., Redmond, L. S., Salomon, I., Collantes, G. O. and Choo, S. (2004) When is commuting desirable to the individual? *Growth and Change*, 35(3) pp. 334–359.

Peters, D. (2013) Going the extra mile. Australian healthcare design, in Copeland, K. ed., *Australian Healthcare Design 2005–2015: A Critical Review of the Design and Build of Healthcare Infrastructure in Australia*, International Academy for Design and Health, Brisbane.

Schoeppe, S., Tranter, P., Duncan, M. J., Curtis, C., Carver, A. and Malone, K. (2016) Australian children's independent mobility levels: Secondary analyses of cross-sectional data between 1991 and 2012. *Children's Geographies*, 14(4) pp. 408–421.

Standing Committee on Public Works (2001) *Report: Sick Building Syndrome*, Report No. 52/07. April 2001, NSW Legislative Assembly, Sydney, NSW.

Tucci, J., Mitchell, J. and Goddard, C. (2007) *Modern Children in Australia*. Australian Childhood Foundation, Melbourne.

Ulrich, R. S. (1984) View through a window may influence recovery from surgery. *Science*, 224(4647) pp. 420–421.

Western Australian Department of Sport and Recreation (2011) *Guide to Shared Use Facilities in the Sport and Recreation Community*, Western Australian Department of Sport and Recreation, Leederville, WA.

Whitzman, C. and Pike, L. (2007) *From Battery-Reared to Free Range Children: Institutional Barriers and Enablers to Childrenís Independent Mobility in Victoria, Australia*, Australasian Centre for Governance and Management of Urban Transportation, Melbourne.

11 Reflections on Principles of Healthy Planning

Introduction

We have discussed the way Australia's planning intersects with several Domains of Wellbeing (Part II) and how we can plan for health across a series of Domains of the Built Environment (Part III). The way professional planners and planning researchers practise their respective trades—the principles that guide the decisions they make—also has powerful implications for the health and wellbeing of the Australian community. This final chapter of our book is dedicated to reflections on key principles for guiding healthy planning in Australia.

Presented here is an overview of several concepts that have extensive theoretical and applied histories. Multifaceted matters such as inclusion, diversity, equity and urgency occupy the attention of researchers who consider and apply these concepts with a breadth and depth we cannot hope to emulate. We acknowledge that our brevity will override a degree of the nuance that underpins understandings of urban and health issues. Nevertheless, we propose that the conceptualisations presented here remain helpful in drawing attention to some of the key issues we face in planning Australia's healthy built environments.

Promoting Equity

What Do We Mean by Promoting Equity?

> The route to achieving equity will *not* be accomplished through treating everyone equally. It will be achieved by treating everyone justly according to their circumstances.
>
> (Dressel 2014, emphasis added)

We open with this quote to illustrate the important difference between equality and equity. The distinction will be familiar to health professionals well versed in the thoroughly researched concept of health equity. While equality ensures that everyone has equal access to the resources

Table 11.1 Equality and equity applied in urban planning

Example of equality in urban planning	Example of equity in urban planning
All community consultation is conducted in English because 80% of the population speaks English.	Language translators are present at community consultation projects.
All suburbs have the same number of community gardens, containing the same allotments that are open at the same hours.	There are more community gardens in lower-income neighbourhoods because the population has less access to private yard space and shops selling fresh produce. These gardens have different types of allotments and are open for long hours.

they need to live and flourish in modern life, equity addresses the unique needs of vulnerable populations to ensure equity of outcome as well as equity of access. Two examples of the application of equality compared with equity in urban planning are presented in Table 11.1.

Throughout the last 30 years in Australia, there has been a notable push for our society to accept that the provision of equal access is a reasonable hallmark of a successful modern country. The health outcomes associated with this reveal that the opposite is true. Equal access does not translate into equal outcomes because it fails to acknowledge that people come to the challenges of life with different abilities, skills and resources.

Why Promoting Equity Is Important for Health

Promoting equity is important for health because health disparities display a social gradient. In general, the higher a person's socio-economic position, the healthier he or she is. People from poorer social or economic circumstances have increased rates of illness and disability and live shorter lives than those who are more advantaged. In Australia, this is illustrated by the differences in life expectancies across the nation. In 2016, a man born in remote New South Wales had a life expectancy 13 years less than a man born in the affluent suburb of Mosman in Sydney (Australian Institute of Health and Welfare [AIHW] 2016).

Promoting equity is also important for health because such a focus necessitates a critical review of the common, yet damaging belief that health is the responsibility of the individual. In line with the general neo-liberal ethos that has permeated Australia's governance (explained in detail below), national health policy has drifted towards a focus on individual lifestyle adaptation and curative medical interventions. This is despite the evidence that addressing the social gradient of health has a greater impact on population health than medical interventions (Baum

2018). Many argue that the deferral of responsibility from society to the individual exacerbates the social gradient to ill health by placing the largest burden of responsibility on those who have the least control over their lives (Glasgow and Schrecker 2016). While we perpetuate inequitable access to the environments required for health, the individual remains the target for ineffective interventions and blame.

The third reason that equity is an important principle for healthy planning is because acknowledgement of equity as a common goal provides foundations for the tolerance of difference in other aspects of life. Later in this chapter, we discuss diversity. Australia is an extremely culturally diverse society, and although our policies and attitudes towards cultural differences are imperfect—sometimes even shameful—and always shifting, in many ways, Australia is a success story of cultural diversity. One reason for this is that we have maintained a strong egalitarian ethos. The concept of the 'fair go' is writ large in Australia's social history, and this commitment to equity, although contingent, as described in Chapter 1—Australia and Australia's Planning, provides a platform on which to rationalise cultural differences. If this commitment continues to be eroded by, for example, the positioning of health issues as the sole responsibility of the individual over the state, or by deferring the provision of services to the private market, we risk exposing other tensions and resentments. This final link between equity and health is the least tangible and most difficult to quantify or test. However, it is founded on the evidence-based notion that an equitable society is a more convivial and healthy one.

Box 11.1 Taking responsibility for childhood obesity in Australia

Policies to tackle childhood obesity in Australia often target the individual child or their carer rather than the wider environment. In 2014–2015, just over one in four (26%) Australian children aged five to 14 and nearly four in ten (37%) young people aged 15–24 were overweight or obese. Children and young adults from lower socio-economic backgrounds were more likely to be overweight and obese than others (Australian Institute of Health and Welfare [AIHW] 2016). This is a major concern for the future health of Australians, and as such, childhood obesity has been listed as a priority by several Australian governments. We know that the childhood obesity problem stems not necessarily from a lack of willpower—or greed—on the part of either the child or their carer. People who earn less or are less educated are not necessarily lazier or more gluttonous than the rest of the population. Instead, evidence shows that childhood obesity is the result of social and built environments that promote eating on the run and eating often, using marketing in which energy-dense fast foods are consistently and mercilessly represented as the most appealing, appropriate and cheap options. Lower-income families are less likely to live within walking distance of a well-stocked neighbourhood supermarket, less able to afford the ingredients for an easy-to-make, nutritious home-cooked meal and less likely to have ready access to an attractive space in which to prepare that meal. They are more likely to live in close proximity to a warm, inviting, cheap, familiar, on-demand fast-food outlet. Yet policymakers in Australia continue to shy away from regulation of the fast-food industry by, for example, not moderating fast-food advertising or preventing the co-location of fast-food outlets and schools. Instead, we continue to invest in individually tailored solutions, ranging from nutritional labelling to bariatric surgery. These are interventions that fail to address the problem because they fail to recognise that its true cause is the wider environment, not the individuals left to navigate it.

Planning and Promoting Equity in Australia

To promote equity, we need to define what it is we are seeking to equalise. In the context of health, it is the equitable distribution of the social determinants of health, which we introduced in Chapter 2—Australia's Health. These are the conditions in which people are born, grow, live, work and age. Factors such as income, education, employment, empowerment and social support act to strengthen or undermine health and wellbeing. These circumstances are shaped by the distribution of money, power and resources at global, national and local levels (Wilkinson and Marmot 2003).

In 2008, the World Health Organization published a report of the Commission on the Social Determinants of Health (Marmot et al. 2008). Headed by the world's most respected voice on social determinants of health, Sir Michael Marmot, the aim of the commission was to review evidence and recommend policies to improve the health of vulnerable populations around the world. It had a distinct focus on turning public health knowledge into political action. In leading this commission, Marmot declared that "health should be of concern to policymakers in every sector, not solely those involved in health policy" (Marmot 2005, p. 1099). This is an open invitation to urban planners to adopt health, including health equity, as a planning responsibility.

Australian planners are well versed in the fundamentals of planning the equitable city. Our planners have access to the data and the grounded knowledge required to expose gaps in the provision of services. For example, a local infrastructure planner can readily identify the communities that do not have internet broadband access but need it. A facilities planner working at the State Department of Education has information ready to hand to prepare a geographical analysis of the at-capacity schools across a city and forecast those that will soon need to be extended. A transport planner working for Sydney's City Rail knows all too well which train service is unreliable and which train station is routinely missed during the peak because of overcrowding. Australia's planners also have the skills and insights to raise concerns about shortages in the provision of residential stock before such shortages create the kind of housing affordability crises we have seen recently in some of the nation's largest cities. Furthermore, based on our combined experience working both as and with planners, we believe strongly that the Australian planning profession values equity as a normative criterion.

The real challenge for planners promoting equity in Australia is the need to operate within the constraints of the nation's dominant political economy. Put simply, this means the way systems of production and trade (the economy) are related to prevailing trends of law, custom and government. In Australia today, we have a neo-liberal system, epitomised by "the subjugation of the public to the private, the state to the market, the social to the economic" (Clarke 2004, p. 4). This system has been enforced since the latter half of the 20th Century—a period symbolised by the introduction of economic rationalist policies and the progressive withdrawal of government intervention in many areas. In painting this picture of free-market audacity, we acknowledge that the practice of land use planning in Australia is not entirely subservient to the market. Regulatory and strategic land use planning remains an important institution for the setting and implementation of decision-making frameworks, often enshrined in statutory documents. This intention, however, runs counter to prevailing political and social conditions, which tend to value market efficiency over land use regulation (Manning-Thomas 2015). As a result, while we may not have an entirely neo-liberal planning system in Australia, the systems within which planning operates are, increasingly, neo-liberal.

By analysing the political, social and economic processes underpinning several episodes of strategic planning in Sydney, we have worked with public health and planning scholars to develop several recommendations for Australian planners seeking to promote health within the often unsupportive confines of a neo-liberal system (Kent et al. 2017). The first is to harness the power of human health's emotive appeal. Relative to other planning concerns, such as environmental sustainability, health is an issue that appeals more directly to the individual. In Chapter 5—Planning for Social Interaction—we introduced the Hofstede model of national cultures. This model suggests that Australia is a highly individual nation, meaning that many of us (but not all) hold concerns for the individual over concerns for the collective good. By making clear the links between good planning principles and human health, planners can leverage this emotion to promote concepts that might otherwise be ignored in developer-driven agendas. The protection of green open spaces for physical activity and community connection is a good example. These are resources that are increasingly in demand for more lucrative uses, such as residential development. By pointing out how important these things are for human health, urban planners can make a compelling and robust case for their preservation.

A second way planning for health can leverage space in a neo-liberal system is by speaking the language of the market. In 2014–2015, Australia spent $162 billion on health (AIHW 2016). This expenditure increases from year to year, faster than the growth rates for inflation, the population or the economy. Treatments for the chronic non-communicable diseases featured throughout this book are expensive, and their prevention would result in considerable cost savings to both the Australian government and individuals. These savings can be captured in decision-making tools such as cost-benefit analyses. This will only occur, however, if the true costs of *not* providing healthy built environment infrastructure are recognised across the board. At present, this is not the case in Australia. The relatively siloed government departments of health, transport and urban planning operate to different budgetary timeframes and agendas. Planners are in a powerful position to work together with public health professionals to develop a deeper understanding of the cost savings to health of better urban planning decisions and to promote the use of robust and comprehensive cost-benefit analyses in decision-making.

Finally, health can be promoted in a neo-liberal system by harnessing the power of the health fraternity. Australian research shows that often it is the voice of a well-versed and respected individual that can make the difference when it comes to preserving a piece of open space, funding a cycleway or protecting the use of land for farmers markets (Harris et al. 2017). Health professionals are held in high esteem in Australia. Each year, polling company Roy Morgan conducts an Image of Professions Survey, asking Australians to rank 30 professions by characteristics such as ethics and honesty. Medical professionals, such as nurses, doctors, pharmacists and dentists, consistently feature in the top five (Roy Morgan Research 2017). This indicates that the voices of these professionals are trusted, potentially making them influential spokespeople for healthy built environment agendas.

This chapter has so far discussed the importance of equity as a planning principle. We opened by describing the differences between equity and equality. Equity addresses the unique needs of vulnerable populations to ensure equity of outcome as well as equity of access. This obviously requires meaningful engagement with diversity, which is the subject of the next section.

Incorporating Diversity

What Do We Mean by Incorporating Diversity? A Step Beyond Acknowledgement

The foundations of diversity in modern life are innumerable. In Australia, we all come to live in urban spaces from different backgrounds, experiences and understandings, and we all have individual preferences. These things are shaped by age, gender, ability, sexual orientation, level of education, income, religious and political beliefs, Indigeneity and ethnicity, to name a few. Of course, these markers of diversity are not exclusive, often interacting and shifting through time and space.

This diversity offers countless opportunities. Indeed, diversity is a crucial component of a healthy society. Yet diversity can also become the basis for tension. To maximise the benefits of diversity and manage the conflicts that inevitably arise, diversity needs to be incorporated genuinely into ways of doing, being and knowing in contemporary Australian society. This is not just about acknowledging that we have our differences. It is about welcoming them, encouraging them, including them and ultimately seeking to understand them. There are some indicators suggesting that this is not currently the case in Australia.

We have already mentioned in Chapter 5—Planning for Social Interaction—the concern that Australia's societal connections are becoming more bounded by our own networks. We rely less and less on incidental interactions with the neighbours, fellow travellers and others with whom we cross paths to provide us with a sense of connection and belonging. Instead, connections are increasingly based on existing networks—common interest groups, work colleagues or friends of friends. The social media giant Facebook is a perfect illustration of this. Our Facebook network is first determined by us during the act of requesting and accepting friends. It then grows through degrees of separation unpicked and minimised by algorithms that corral a group of people who are relative strangers, yet still display similar tastes, backgrounds, beliefs and skills. Our newsfeed, the advertisements we see, suggestions for friends, events, objects and groups, are all bounded by the cyber fence of our browsing histories. This is a system of networking augmented time and time again through platforms far less sophisticated than Facebook. It is a phenomenon enhanced by technology that provides both the platform for interactions and the excuse to avoid even eye contact with those around us. This relatively new way of relating poses several threats to the incorporation of diversity into our lives—if we are blind to those immediately around us, we miss their differences. Our skills to learn, accommodate, shift, question and resolve differences become either diminished or do not develop.

People are at the heart of diversity. However, when we refer to incorporating diversity for health, we are not only talking about people. There are also diverse ways of knowing and doing things, which, if translated, understood and adapted, can push the boundaries of knowledge and practice in directions that promote health. We are particularly interested in the need for the healthy built environments agenda in Australia to accommodate different ways of knowing, or epistemologies. As planning professionals working amongst respected colleagues from public health, we have been exposed to, and needed to engage with, new epistemologies. For example, the health profession has an established standard of evidence with roots in clinical epidemiology. Evidence-based medicine (EBM) classifies evidence by its strength. It deems that sound recommendations for interventions can only come from the strongest types of evidence, classified as meta-analyses, systematic reviews and randomised controlled trials. Urban planning decisions are very rarely made on the basis of this kind of quantitative evidence. Australian urban planning's early to mid-20th Century focus on green belt cities, for example, was based on an historical appreciation of the health benefits of open space for overcrowded and dirty cities. Schemes such as Sydney's *County of Cumberland Plan* (1951) and Perth's *Endowment Lands Act* (1920) reflect this appreciation. There are many reasons, both historical and epistemological, for this way of thinking about the evidence required to justify policy change. This does not mean that urban planning is somehow a less competent or rigorous profession.

An important factor behind the different ways health and built environment professions come to the challenge of healthy built environments is unrelated to epistemology—rather, it is a reflection of the nature of the problem. The kind of evidence required by paradigms such as EBM simply cannot be generated for the way people live and move around built environments. Our cities are not machines that can be quantified and observed from a dashboard. Even with the availability of big data that has recently excited many research agendas, some situations will only be understood by observing, listening, recording and synthesising the perceptions and practices of real people. By incorporating different ways of thinking about evidence, including increased appreciation of qualitative data, more realistic recommendations for policy and behavioural change can replace the common calls for causal proof that conclude so many journal articles in this space.

Why Is Incorporating Diversity Important for Health?

> Across all Biosystems, diversity is a source of strength
>
> (*Mackay 2018*, p. 81).

Although difference is usually at the heart of tension in a society, it is also a source of great strength. According to the very biological 'insurance hypothesis', genetic diversity of plants, animals and other living organisms "insures ecosystems against declines in their functioning because many species provide greater guarantees that some will maintain functioning even if others fail" (Yachi and Loreau 1999, p. 1463). Applying this theory to not only genetic diversity but also a multiplicity of ideas, structures and ways of doing things in our cities, diversity is unquestionably the central requisite for resilience through processes of change. Furthermore, it is only by experiencing diversity that we can learn to question, and resolve, differences. At a very innate and personal level, experiences of diversity stimulate the development of greater cognitive flexibility, which, in psychological literature, is identified as a fundamental skill for human survival (Crisp and Turner 2011). Diversity is therefore critical to individual and societal health because it provides an insurance plan for resilience as well as the opportunity for individuals to hone skills of adaptation.

Diversity Prompts an Appreciation of Context

We are not only interested in diversity because of its role as both insurance policy and teacher. From a healthy planning perspective, the ultimate benefit of incorporating diversity concerns into planning is that it prompts us to acknowledge and explore context.

Healthy built environment research and practice must prioritise consideration of the 'subtleties of diversity' (Evans 2009, p. 199)—a recurring theme throughout this book. By this, we simply mean that in transferring the lessons learnt from one built environment to another, the unique elements of each component, as well as the various constructs of the whole, must be known and considered. What works to promote health in one locality or within a particular social group will not necessarily work elsewhere.

Our interest in context stems firstly from the fact that we, as planners, are genuinely bewildered by the preoccupation of some research on health determinants with establishing common measures, transferable interventions and causal proof for healthy built environments. It is as though the diverse and shifting cultural, social, biophysical, political, economic and historical elements that make up a place are considered no more heterogeneous than one human cell is to the next. Governance of the built environment is contested—economic, political and popular agendas must be pieced together alongside scientific evidence to bring about change.

Acknowledging contextuality in relation to healthy built environment research and practice must not be viewed as an impediment. Too often, the things that count (to researchers, policymakers and practitioners) are simply those that can be counted. The issues that really matter are ignored because they are too difficult to quantify or measure. Complexity needs to be taken seriously in both the application of research to policy and the design of future research agendas. There are various ways to achieve this that we now consider.

Firstly, we are lucky in Australia to have access to a wealth of resources that can be mined to build a picture of a community or issue. We have attempted to corral some of these into Appendix Two. Resources have no doubt been missed or developed since the time of writing, and we urge our readers to think laterally about the types of data that might be available to fill the complex gaps left by a true consideration of context.

Secondly, we promote the use of mixed methods research techniques. In the healthy built environment space, this often means introducing qualitative techniques to quantitative data analysis. It is amazing what can be revealed to a researcher or practitioner simply by respectful and targeted observations of the people and places comprising a practice or place. There is not the space here to review the array of qualitative methods available to assist in unpicking the complexity of context. In-depth interviews, focus groups, discourse analysis, photo diary research, walking interviews and other ethnographic methods are all techniques for understanding that are increasingly used in healthy built environment research in Australia. We applaud this.

Thirdly, there are several safeguards required to progress work towards a more situated, qualitative and comprehensive approach to healthy built environment research and practice in Australia. Of course, methods should be entirely transparent and situated within the existing research agenda. Case study research should be made available in both scholarly publications and other easily accessible repositories. Finally, at all times, researchers must engender respect and trust within the Australian community.

Planning and Incorporating Diversity in Australia

Urban planning in Australia has a pivotal role to play in incorporating diversity in a way that promotes health. To demonstrate this, we have chosen to focus our discussion on the opportunities and threats presented by cultural diversity, shining a particular spotlight on immigrants from overseas countries settling in Australia.

Details on the cultural make-up of modern Australia are outlined in Chapter 1—Australia and Australia's Planning. In short, four decades after the end of the shameful White Australia policy, in the context of Australian immigration, multicultural diversity is now well established. In 2016, just over 26% of Australia's population were immigrants (defined as born in a country other than Australia). This is one of the highest rates of all Organization for Economic Co-operation and Development (OECD) countries. Even more interesting is that one in five of these new residents arrived in the five years preceding 2016.

In the context of this unique cultural diversity, Australia has not escaped the rising tide of anti-immigration sentiment that has recently swept many OECD countries. At the time of writing, there is increasing popular support for right-wing, anti-immigrant, anti-refugee parties across Europe. In the United States, President Donald Trump maintains his promise to build a wall to stop Mexican immigration and is in pursuit of deportation of those already residing illegally. In Australia, we have Senator Pauline Hanson of the right-wing party One Nation advocating for a ban on further Muslim immigration. Meanwhile, the Australian government's appalling policy of turning back asylum seeker boats and depositing 'boat people'—including children—into offshore detention centres continues and is a contested political and social issue.

It is reassuring to note, however, that public support for immigration in Australia has recently increased considerably, and that this increase is actually in line with the rise in immigration levels. The Scanlon Foundation was established in 2001 to act as a driver of research on social cohesion in Australia. Each year, the foundation (in conjunction with Monash University and the Australian Multicultural Foundation) undertakes one or more surveys on social cohesion. Their data shows that when immigration intakes in the early 1990s were the lowest since the post-war immigration program began, between two-thirds and three-quarters of Australians surveyed reported they thought immigration was 'too high'. Yet, by 2015, 60% thought immigration intake levels were 'just right'. This is a doubling of support over the past two decades (Markus 2016).

Public opposition to particular cohorts of immigrants is, sadly, a different matter. In 1981, an analysis from Macquarie University (New South Wales) reported that 48% of Australians thought there were too many Asian immigrants arriving in Australia (Collins 2016). Attitudes towards immigrants from Asia have since softened; however, attitudes towards those from Iraq and Lebanon have replaced this disdain. A recent study found that one in ten Australians is 'highly Islamophobic' and has a fear of Muslims (Markus 2016).

It seems that while diversity is integral to individual health and the functioning of society, diversity can be a precursor to tension. It is in the task of preventing the emergence of tensions in our communities, and allaying them should they arise, that urban planning can shine.

Firstly, good planning gives people a voice. Community consultation and collaboration are oft-repeated tenets of urban planning in Australia, yet countless studies provide evidence that the Australian public do not feel as though they have a say in the way their environment is planned and managed (see, for example, Burton 2017). This sense of exclusion, or disenfranchisement, from the public consultation elements of Australia's urban planning systems is amplified for minority groups.

Secondly, good planning encourages tension-free day-to-day interactions. We have touched on this in detail in Chapter 5—Planning for Social Interaction. Convivial interactions occur in public spaces that are not overcrowded, easy to use and embellished with 'talking points'— places to talk and things to talk about.

Thirdly, good planning enables our built environments to mirror diversity. There are multiple examples of intentional dedications to the different cultures that make up Australia's urban areas. These are, of course, important. Yet a true appreciation of difference is not fostered simply by a work of public art. It arises when our residential streetscapes are allowed to be diverse. An appreciation of diversity is fostered when our streetscapes can evolve organically, our retail spaces can genuinely support mixed uses and the spaces in between are adaptable to the requirements, preferences and sometimes simple whims of multiplicity. Difference is silenced by narrow and prescriptive design guidelines. Business experimentation is curtailed through strict requirements for long-term lease agreements, signage and permissible uses. The use of open space is inhibited by the ideas and preferences of a particular dominant political economy. A genuine audit would reveal many policies used by planners that inadvertently prevent our urban environments from mirroring the rich and realistic diversity that is the Australian population.

Finally, planners can also contribute to diversity by working together with other disciplines. We have already discussed the need for urban planning and health professionals to establish mutual understandings of key concepts such as evidence and policy development. Education is crucial in working towards this mutuality. We have been instrumental in facilitating interdisciplinary education and awareness of healthy built environments amongst both the health and planning professions. Susan has been particularly active in the development of Australia's first healthy planning tertiary subjects (Thompson and Capon 2010), and we have both presented workshops on the planning system to health professionals, enabling them to take this learning back into the workplace.

Slowing Down in a Speeded-Up World

What Do We Mean by Slowing Down?

The default interpretation of slowing down in the context of urban environments is pejorative. To slow is interpreted as to be backward, lazy or somehow obstructed. Yet slowness can also imply deliberation, enabling attention to detail, thoughtfulness and the exercise of care.

The 'acceleration of just about everything' is a common observation in modern life (Gleick 2000). The way we work, travel, communicate, consume, love, discard, decide and distrust are all now shaped by an overwhelming pressure for speed. And the rate of this acceleration itself is also increasing. Nothing seems to stay the same for very long, and if we are caught out doing just that, many of us are consumed by shame or fear—of missing out, falling back or fading into obsolescence. German sociologist Hartmut Rosa calls this 'social acceleration' (Rosa 2003). In his landmark paper of that title, he defines three components to social acceleration.

Technological Acceleration

The acceleration of technology is the most obvious evidence of our speeded-up world. Technology has indeed transformed the way we live—from the automation of previously manual tasks to the accomplishment of new tasks that make up modern life in the internet age. The relative contemporary speeds of communication, transport and exchange are illustrative cases.

Acceleration of Social Change

Social change refers to the dynamism of social and cultural institutions and practices. Rosa describes contemporary social acceleration as dynamism. It is epitomised by rapidly shifting attitudes, values, fashions and lifestyles. In Australia, this dynamism is reflected in our political leadership, which in recent times has become more aggressive and less consistent.

Personal Acceleration

The third type of social acceleration refers to the speed and compression of actions and experiences in everyday life. These are both subjective and objective phenomena (although, as always, we advise these are never exclusive). Subjectively, personal acceleration is reflected in self-reported experiences of time scarcity or acknowledgements of the sense of rush and busyness that pervades modern life. Objectively, personal acceleration can be measured by examination of the time dedicated to certain tasks and the time spent undertaking multiple tasks simultaneously. Although this is undoubtedly a global phenomenon, there is Australian evidence that we are eating more quickly, sleeping less and speaking at a more rapid pace when compared with our ancestors (ABS 2006). This concept of personal acceleration is intriguing in the context of the technological acceleration mentioned above. Technological innovation implies a decrease in the amount of time required to accomplish the demands of daily life. This should result in an increase in free time, which would result in personal deceleration. However, the data suggests that Australia is not a society sitting with abundant spare time. Instead, any time that is freed up is quickly filled by an insatiable drive to accomplish more in less time.

It is beyond the scope of this book to review the processes at work in speeding up our world. We acknowledge that the desire to get ahead and not 'miss out' is quite simply an innate biological drive to survive. What seems amiss in our society is that this obsession with speed and ambition has rendered us blind to the long-term perspective required to experience our longer life expectancies. We are now living longer but increasingly thinking and acting only in the moment. The health impacts of these trends, and the health benefits of their arrest, are now discussed.

Why Is Slowing Down Important for Health?

There are multiple pathways between health and time. For the individual, slowing down is an opportunity to etch out the space and time needed to be healthy. For planners and others responsible for land use decision-making in Australia, slowing down enables proper consideration of the stakeholders and situations that characterise our built environments. The following section will focus on both these individual and societal benefits of slowing down.

Individuals Slowing Down

The effectiveness of healthy built environments relies on individuals having time- whether it is time to go for a walk, to explore a neighbourhood and meet new people or to perfect a new cooking routine that is healthier but takes slightly longer than an online take-away order. As intimated above, time in modern life is a scarce resource, and data from the Australian Bureau of Statistics confirms this is this case. The most recent Time Use Survey was completed in 2006. It showed that between 1997 and 2006, the proportion of Australians aged 15 years and older who often or always felt rushed or pressed for time increased from 35% to 45%. The HILDA survey also asked respondents how often they felt rushed or pressed for time. Leading a team of scholars primarily from the Australian National University, Lyndall Strazdins used this data to position time as a social determinant of health (Strazdins et al. 2016). The research confirmed an increase in Australians self-reporting a feeling of rush, linking this to poorer self-reported mental and physical health. Strazdins also demonstrated a link between feeling rushed and lower socio-economic status. This suggests that the acceleration of daily life has health impacts not only because it limits the capacity of the individual but also because it has shifted the various structures that determine this capacity.

Societal Slowing

The notion of time as a social determinant of health prompts focus on the way social acceleration affects the practice of healthy planning. From a societal perspective, the temporal scales of capital growth and political cycles (which are undeniably related) clash regularly with those required to facilitate a considered evaluation of the way forward for our cities. Qualitative research confirms that planners in Australia rarely have the time required to apply their expertise in healthy built environments (McCosker et al. 2018). New innovations, trends, risks and benefits come and go with such rapidity that it is impossible to give due consideration to the complexity of built environment matters that affect human health. And no matter how supposedly 'efficient' our planners and planning systems become, it is inevitable that the timetable of the market will be faster and less predictable than is required by best practice planning, including planning for health. The speed of the planning and development system is therefore a key risk for healthy planning in Australia.

Planning and Slowing Down Australia

We have seen some movements—many of them global—towards the appreciation of 'slow'. The slow food movement and the concept of slow cycling are examples (Tranter 2012). Yet slowness is a luxury in modern life. This is confirmed in Australian research by Strazdins et al. (2016), which proves that time pressures are socially and economically patterned, impacting the wealthy less than the poor. This section addresses how urban planning in Australia might work towards redressing this.

In Chapter 4—Planning for Physical Activity—we describe the way time can be a proxy for motivation. Applying this premise, feeling rushed might contribute to poor health because it erodes an individual's capacity, self-belief and enjoyment of healthier ways of living. Good urban planning can increase personal motivation. It can ensure that the conditions for healthy behaviours are readily accessible, safe and attractive. These conditions, and recommendations for their proper planning for health, have filled the pages of this book.

In addition to increasing motivation, good urban planning can return some time to the Australian families and individuals desperately crying out for 'a break'. Implementation of the decisions planners make can reduce the time people in cities spend commuting. We can try to minimise distances between land uses so that the demands of being a good parent, carer or friend can be satisfied in less time.

The fact that our society tends to fill each spare minute with yet more activity suggests that a reduction in travel time itself will not be enough to slow down our speeded-up world—nor will it be sufficient to elicit health benefits. We, as planners, cannot put the brakes on the endless cycle of economic growth and individual and collective advancement implied by the countless agendas determining the fate of the modern world. In both Australia and globally, it is a reality that planning is more often left to mop up, or accommodate, the unintended consequences of an over-reliance on a market-driven political economy.

To truly push forward with making our cities, and lives, healthier, we assert the need not only to operate within the inevitable constraints of this seemingly undying commitment to growth but also to take any opportunity we can to question it. We have outlined above that human health is an emotive and individual issue. Health is, therefore, perhaps better positioned to question the pace of development than some of the agendas that have been used to drive change in the immediate past. Threats to individual health cannot be ignored in the same way that whole-of-society threats, such as climate change, disappearing biodiversity and global inequality are unheeded. By articulating with clarity some of the quite direct pathways between the pace of modern life and individual and societal ill health, we can use this emotion to drive change.

Conclusion

This chapter has been about process. It is included in recognition that the way we approach urban planning for health is just as important as what we plan. Promoting equity, incorporating diversity and slowing down our speeded-up world are all complex concepts, yet they are the processes that define many elements of modern life. We believe that a better understanding of these 'backdrops' to behaviours and environments will advance the healthy built environment agenda in Australia and elsewhere. It will move us forward from our sometimes unhelpful preoccupation with design outcomes.

This is the final chapter in *Planning Australia's Healthy Built Environments*. The ever-present message from our work is that so many of our recommendations rely on a return to equity as a key driver of urban planning decision-making. Quite simply, this means the (re)prioritisation of wellbeing over economic growth. This is a crucial barrier to planning Australia's healthy built environments. Yet, while it is a barrier, it is not insurmountable. Indeed, key to its transcendence may well be harnessing the power of health as a significant concern for all.

References

Australian Bureau of Statistics (2006) *How Australians Use Their Time*, Cat. no. 4153.0, Australian Bureau of Statistics, Canberra, www.abs.gov.au [Accessed 29 June 2018].

Australian Institute of Health and Welfare (2016) *Australia's Health 2016*, Australian Institute of Health and Welfare, Canberra.

Baum, F. (2018) People's health and the social determinants of health. *Health Promotion Journal of Australia*, 29(1) pp. 8–9.

Burton, P. (2017) Is Urban planning in Australia hindered by poor metropolitan governance? *Urban Science*, 1(4) p. 34.

Clarke, J. (2004) Consumerism and the remaking of state-citizen relationships, in Marston, G. and McDonald, C. eds., *Analysing Social Policy: A Governmental Approach*, Edward Elgar Publishing, Brighton.

Collins, J. (2016) Perspectives on migrants distorted by politics of prejudice. *The Conversation*, 20 September 2006, http://theconversation.com/ [Accessed 1 May 2018].

Crisp, R. J. and Turner, R. N. (2011) Cognitive adaptation to the experience of social and cultural diversity. *Psychological Bulletin*, 137(2) pp. 242–266.

Dressel, P. (2014) *Racial Equality or Racial Equity? The Difference it Makes*, Race Matters Institute, 2 April, http://viablefuturescenter.org/racemattersinstitute/2014/04/02/racial-equality-or-racial-equity-the-difference-it-makes/ [Accessed 13 June 2018].

Evans, S. (2009) 'That lot up there and us down here': Social interaction and a sense of community in a mixed tenure UK retirement village. *Ageing and Society*, 29(2) pp. 199–216.

Glasgow, S. and Schrecker, T. (2016) The double burden of neo-liberalism? Non-communicable disease policies and the global political economy of risk. *Health and Place*, 39 pp. 204–211.

Gleick, J. (2000) *Faster: The Acceleration of Just About Everything*, Pantheon Books, New York.

Harris, P., Kent, J., Sainsbury, P., Marie-Thow, A., Baum, F., Friel, S. and McCue, P. (2017) Creating 'healthy built environment' legislation in Australia: A policy analysis. *Health Promotion International* pp. 1–11. doi:10.1093/heapro/dax055.

Kent, J. L., Harris, P., Sainsbury, P., Baum, F., McCue, P. and Thompson, S. (2017) Influencing Urban planning policy: An exploration from the perspective of public health. *Urban Policy and Research*, 36(1) pp. 20–34.

Mackay, H. (2018) *Australia Reimagined: Towards a More Compassionate, Less Anxious Society*, Pan McMillan, Sydney, NSW.

Manning-Thomas, J. (2015) The minority-race planner in the quest for the just city. *Planning Theory*, 7(3) pp. 227–247.

Markus, A. (2016) *Australians Today: The Australia@2015 Scanlon Foundation Survey*, The Scanlon Foundation, Melbourne.

Marmot, M. (2005) Social determinants of health inequalities. *The Lancet*, 365(9464) pp. 1099–1104.

Marmot, M., Friel, S., Bell, R., Houweling, T. A. and Taylor, S. (2008) Closing the gap in a generation: Health equity through action on the social determinants of health. *The Lancet* 372(9650) pp. 1661–1669.

McCosker, A., Matan, A. and Marinova, D. (2018) Policies, politics, and paradigms: Healthy planning in Australian local government. *Sustainability*, 10(4) p. 1008.

Rosa, H. (2003) Social acceleration: Ethical and political consequences of a desynchronized high–speed society. *Constellations*, 10(1) pp. 3–33.

Roy Morgan Research (2017) *Image of Professions Survey 2017: Health Professionals Continue Domination with Nurses Most Highly Regarded Again: Followed by Doctors and Pharmacists*. Roy Morgan Research, 7 June 2017, www.roymorgan.com/findings/7244-roy-morgan-image-of-professions-may-2017-201706051543 [Accessed 13 June 2018].

Strazdins, L., Welsh, J., Korda, R., Broom, D. and Paolucci, F. (2016) Not all hours are equal: Could time be a social determinant of health? *Sociology of Health and Illness*, 38(1) pp. 21–42.

Thompson, S. M. and Capon, A. G. (2010) Designing a Healthy and Sustainable Future: A vision for interdisciplinary education, research and leadership. *Proceedings of ConnectED 2010*, 2nd International Conference on Design Education, 28 June to 1 July 2010, UNSW, Sydney, NSW.

Tranter, P. J. (2012) Effective speed: Cycling because it's "Faster", in Pucher, J. and Buehler, R. eds., *City Cycling*, MIT Press, Cambridge, MA.

Wilkinson, R. G. and Marmot, M. (2003) *Social Determinants of Health: The Solid Facts*, 2nd edition, World Health Organization, Copenhagen.

Yachi, S. and Loreau, M. (1999) Biodiversity and ecosystem productivity in a fluctuating environment: The insurance hypothesis. *Proceedings of the National Academy of Sciences*, 96(4) pp. 1463–1468.

Appendix One

Glossary

The list below covers some of the terms used in this book that may be unfamiliar to readers outside Australia. For a list of healthy planning terms, we recommend our readers consult the glossary associated with the Heart Foundation's Healthy Active by Design initiative. The text *Making Healthy Places*, edited by Dannenberg et al. (2011), also contains a comprehensive glossary of healthy planning terms. Both of these fantastic resources are described in Appendix Two.

Term	Description
Active transport	Walking, cycling or using a push scooter.
Alternative transport	Any transport mode alternative to the private car including walking, cycling, public transport, and commercial and peer-to-peer car sharing.
Australian census	The census in Australia, officially known as the Census of Population and Housing. This is a count of the population of Australia on one night, held every five years. Participation in the census is compulsory.
BMX	An abbreviation for bicycle motocross, which is a cycle sport performed on BMX bikes on- or off-road for recreation and competition.
Bushwalking	The Australian word for hiking, which involves walking through undeveloped land or wilderness on tracks or cross-country through the Australian bush.
Commonwealth	In Australia, the term 'Commonwealth' is used to refer to the Commonwealth of Australia as a nation and Australia's membership of the group known as the Commonwealth of Nations. This is an intergovernmental organisation of 53 member States that are mostly former territories of the British Empire.

Term	Description
Community garden	Any piece of land gardened by a group of people. In Australia, community gardens are usually on public land and are gardened to provide fresh produce and plants. They are publicly functioning in terms of ownership, access and management and are typically owned in trust by Local government organisations.
Joint- or shared-use agreement	An arrangement between a school (usually at the discretion of the school's Principal) and community to share facilities. This might mean opening up a hall on the school grounds for an evening drawing class (shared use) or the more complex option where facilities are actually planned, built and managed by both a school and a partner organisation (joint use).
Long Boom	A term used to describe a series of economic, demographic and technological changes associated with the 1950s and 1960s. This was a defining period of political stability, economic prosperity and unprecedented population growth in Australia.
Peri-urban area	An area immediately adjoining an urban area, situated on the periphery of large towns and cities.
Socio-Economic Indexes for Areas (SEIFA)	An index developed by the Australian Bureau of Statistics that ranks geographical areas in Australia according to relative socio-economic advantage and disadvantage. The indexes are based on information from the Australian census. Higher scores reflect lower levels of disadvantage.
Strata Title	In Australia, Strata Title governs the majority of apartments and other forms of attached dwellings, such as townhouses. Strata Title allows for separate ownership of each apartment within a building and governance through a 'body corporate' consisting of property owners. The New South Wales State government was the first to introduce the concept in 1961. It has since been adopted nationally across Australia and internationally.
Surf Life Saving	A term used to describe both voluntary lifeguard services and a competitive surf sport. Surf Life Saving Australia is the custodian of both services and sport.
Talking point	Talking points are both places for talking and things to talk about. Talking points are key components of healthy built environments because they facilitate interactions.
Urban agriculture	Growing plants and raising animals on land that has been modified by built form for the primary purpose of food supply, distinguished from rural agriculture by integration into the urban ecological system.

References

Dannenberg, A. L., Frumkin, H. and Jackson, R. J. (2011) *Making Healthy Places: Designing and Building for Health, Well-Being, and Sustainability*, Island Press, London.

Healthy Active by Design (2018) *Glossary*, www.healthyactivebydesign.com.au/glossary [Accessed 15 August 2018].

Appendix Two

Four of Four: Further Information

In writing this book, we have intentionally avoided the prescription of specific design advice. This is because we believe that context should always guide decision-making when planning healthy built environments. This simply means taking into account the circumstances in which plans are made and interventions employed. What works for one neighbourhood/city/State may be inappropriate for another. Of course, there are some basic standards and indicators that can be consulted as a starting point. And if this is what is required, then there is an increasingly large body of research and reporting to consult. Below, we present key sources that we believe may be helpful. The lists are by no means exhaustive; however, they cover useful texts, websites, scholarly journals and data sources. We present four of each.

Four Texts

1. *Creating Healthy Neighborhoods: Evidence-Based Planning and Design Strategies* by Ann Forsyth, Emily Salomon and Laura Smead Chicago, IL: American Planning Association, 250 pages 2017 ISBN: 978–1611901917 (pbk)
2. *The Routledge Handbook of Planning for Health and Well-Being: Shaping a sustainable and healthy future* Edited by Hugh Barton, Susan Thompson, Sarah Burgess, Marcus Grant Abingdon, Oxon; New York, NY: Routledge, 618 pages 2015 ISBN: 978–1138049079 (pbk)
3. *Healthy City Planning: From Neighbourhood to National Health Equity* Jason Corburn Abingdon, Oxon; New York, NY: Routledge, 192 pages 2013 ISBN: 9780415613026 (pbk)
4. *Making Healthy Places: Designing and Building for Health, Well-being, and Sustainability* Edited by Andrew L. Dannenberg, Howard Frumkin, and Richard J. Jackson Washington, DC: Island Press, 440 pages 2011ISBN: 978–1597267274 (pbk)

Four Scholarly Journals

1. *Health and Place* "an interdisciplinary journal dedicated to the study of all aspects of health and healthcare in which place or location matters" Elsevier ISSN: 1353–8292 (online)
2. *Cities and Health* "an innovative new international platform for consolidating research and know-how for city development to support human health". Taylor and Francis ISSN: 2374–8834 (print)
3. *Transport and Health* "devoted to research on the many interactions between transport and health". Elsevier ISSN: 2214–1405 (online)
4. *Urban Policy and Research* "an international journal dedicated to the publication of refereed articles in English in the field of urban studies and urban policy for those with an interest in Australia, New Zealand and the wider Asia Pacific region". Taylor and Francis ISSN: 0811–1146 (print)

Four Websites With Guidelines

1. Healthy Active by Design (Australia) www.healthyactivebydesign. com.au
2. Active Living Research (USA) www.activelivingresearch.org
3. Spatial Planning for Health (UK) www.gov.uk/government/ publications/spatial-planning-for-health-evidence-review
4. Project for Public Spaces (USA) www.pps.org

Four Australian Data Sources

1. Australian Bureau of Statistics: "Australia's national statistical agency, providing trusted official statistics on a wide range of economic, social, population and environmental matters of importance to Australia". www.abs.gov.au
2. Australian Institute of Health and Welfare: Australia's Health "Australia's leading health and welfare statistics agency". www.aihw.gov. au
3. The Household, Income and Labour Dynamics in Australia (HILDA) Survey: "a household-based panel study that collects valuable information about economic and personal wellbeing, labour market dynamics and family life". https://melbourneinstitute.unimelb.edu. au/hilda
4. Profile ID: A commercial organisation using Australian census and other data to provide statistical analysis and data-representation services. https://profile.id.com.au

Index

Note: page numbers in *italic* indicate a figure, page numbers in **bold** indicate a table and underlined page numbers indicate a box on the corresponding page. Note information is denoted with and note number following the page number.